NO LONGER PROPERTY OF
SEATTLE PUBLIC LIBRARY

Green Kids, Sage Families

D1024174

Green Kids, Sage Families

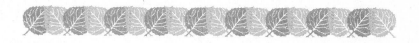

*The Ultimate Guide
to Raising Your
Organic Kids*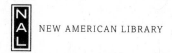

Lynda Fassa

NAL | NEW AMERICAN LIBRARY

New American Library
Published by New American Library, a division of
Penguin Group (USA) Inc., 375 Hudson Street,
New York, New York 10014, USA
Penguin Group (Canada), 90 Eglinton Avenue East, Suite 700, Toronto,
Ontario M4P 2Y3, Canada (a division of Pearson Penguin Canada Inc.)
Penguin Books Ltd., 80 Strand, London WC2R 0RL, England
Penguin Ireland, 25 St. Stephen's Green, Dublin 2,
Ireland (a division of Penguin Books Ltd.)
Penguin Group (Australia), 250 Camberwell Road, Camberwell, Victoria 3124,
Australia (a division of Pearson Australia Group Pty. Ltd.)
Penguin Books India Pvt. Ltd., 11 Community Centre, Panchsheel Park,
New Delhi - 110 017, India
Penguin Group (NZ), 67 Apollo Drive, Rosedale, North Shore 0632,
New Zealand (a division of Pearson New Zealand Ltd.)
Penguin Books (South Africa) (Pty.) Ltd., 24 Sturdee Avenue,
Rosebank, Johannesburg 2196, South Africa

Penguin Books Ltd., Registered Offices: 80 Strand, London WC2R 0RL, England

First published by New American Library, a division of Penguin Group (USA) Inc.

First Printing, January 2009
1   3   5   7   9   10   8   6   4   2

This book is printed on acid-free, recycled paper.

Copyright © Lynda Fassa, 2009
Foreword copyright © Vanessa L. Williams, 2009
For photo credits see page 255.
All rights reserved

 REGISTERED TRADEMARK—MARCA REGISTRADA

Library of Congress Cataloging-in-Publication Data
Fassa, Lynda.
Green kids, sage families : the ultimate guide to raising your organic kids / Lynda Fassa.
p. cm.
ISBN: 978-0-451-22581-8
1. Organic living.   2. Child rearing.   3. Family.   4. Parent and child.   I. Title.
GF77.F38 2008
649'.1—dc22   2008025384

Set in Adobe Garamond
Designed by Jessica Shatan Heslin/Studio Shatan, Inc.

Printed in the United States of America

Without limiting the rights under copyright reserved above, no part of this publication may be
reproduced, stored in or introduced into a retrieval system, or transmitted, in any form, or by any means
(electronic, mechanical, photocopying, recording, or otherwise), without the prior written permission
of both the copyright owner and the above publisher of this book.

PUBLISHER'S NOTE
Every effort has been made to ensure that the information contained in this book is complete and accurate.
However, neither the publisher nor the author is engaged in rendering professional advice or services to
the individual reader. The ideas, procedures, and suggestions contained in this book are not intended as
a substitute for consulting with your physician. All matters regarding your child's health require
medical supervision. Neither the author nor the publisher shall be liable or responsible for any loss or
damage allegedly arising from any information or suggestion in this book. The opinions expressed in
this book represent the personal views of the author and not of the publisher.

The publisher does not have any control over and does not assume any responsibility for author or
third-party Web sites or their content.

The scanning, uploading, and distribution of this book via the Internet or via any other means without
the permission of the publisher is illegal and punishable by law. Please purchase only authorized
electronic editions, and do not participate in or encourage electronic piracy of copyrighted materials.
Your support of the author's rights is appreciated.

To my wonderful sister, Dawn,
for her boundless love, encourgement
and support

Acknowledgments

I want to thank my beautiful sister, Dawn Bridges; my brilliant and gentle editor, Tracy Bernstein; the inspirational and enlightened Vanessa Williams; and my thoughtful and forward-thinking agents, Brian Dubin, Mel Berger, and Strand Conover at William Morris, without whom I could never have had the resources to collect, process, and collate all this good green information. I also want to express my deep gratitude to all of the people who spend their time and energy looking out for the well-being of our environment. We really are all connected to each other, and together, your choices and mine can make the world a safe haven for our growing kids.

So, finally, I want to thank you for picking up this book, because in it you'll find help to give your children the greatest gift—a healthy life.

Contents

Introduction

Life is beautiful. And every life makes a difference, shifting the balance on the earth. When a child enters the world, everything changes—most especially for you and your family, but ultimately for everyone. Each individual experience reflects the promise for the species as a whole.

Layla, my first child, came out screaming and a purplish blue from the protective waxy vernix coating, not the peaches and cream I expected, but still eye-poppingly beautiful to me. Special. She *mattered*, more than anything else in the world. It's a happy, vivid memory I play in my mind like a much-loved rerun, a favored videocassette so adored you bother to keep the clunky old VCR just so you can watch that particular tape, over and over again. The arrival of my second, in the middle of a dark and stormy New England night, was quiet and stealthy. She appeared like an alien being with shining clear eyes ("eyes that shine like centuries," Paul Simon sings in "Born at the Right Time"). My little Mina brought the magical power to charm and enchant. The OB nurse who had stayed with me through a long and dangerous labor said, "She is the most beautiful baby in the world," and I couldn't have agreed more. My third, Nadia, also appeared at night, but in a rabble-rousing, noisy, honky-tonk event. With a larger cast of characters than an eighties miniseries, it was truly a family affair, complete with claps and guffaws as my husband cut the cord, immediately followed by me ravenously devouring a cold quiche my wonderful mother-in-law sneaked into my hospital bag. (Hey, I was hungry—bringin' those kids in through the vortex is hard work!)

Each child has a unique imprint, meaning and significance. But you already know that. You're a parent.

We are the luckiest of the lot, we moms and dads. Whether your child comes biologically through your body or legally through adoption, the result is the same. The responsibility of nurturing and caring for a child is the greatest joy on earth. Nature has perfectly equipped us to love our most valuable citizens, our very own little VIPs.

From when you're first pregnant to when your teen calls you from the mall's movie theater to say the *Love Bug* revival is sold out so she and her formerly responsible posse of pals have opted instead for *Texas Chainsaw Massacre III*, it is a wild, wild ride, filled with terrifying split-second decisions. Precarious and unpredictable, frightening and fabulous, 24-7, it's the toughest job you'll ever love. And through it all we have one overriding desire, instinct, and raison d'être: to keep our kids safe. Embedded in our hearts is the metronome beating that mantra: protect . . . protect . . . protect. . . .

While that instinct is unchanging, every generation of parents needs to remap the journey to find the best way to keep their children healthy and safe. Today scary thoughts of Club Penguin interlopers and MySpace predators abound. But the truth is, the greatest threat to our children's health and happiness is off-line: It's our environment, from global warming to the air we breathe. It's time to wake up and smell the fair trade coffee. Cancer is the number one disease killer of kids in the U.S. Asthma and autism are rampant and, some recent studies suggest, related to pesticide exposure and other chemicals in our environment. One out of seven American children is clinically obese. Our schools, which work so hard to diligently provide our kids with a bright future, may be harboring common substances that threaten their health, safety, and brainpower today. Potentially toxic chemicals are found in products we're using from cosmetics to air fresheners and especially in many of the foods and drinks marketed to our kids. For the first time in generations, researchers say, our children may not live as long as we do.

So, as we've been hustling along, trying our best to keep it all together, it looks like somewhere we may have made a wrong turn. How do we get back on track? It's time to grab the wheel and get back in the driver's seat. I hope to be like a soft-voiced GPS, helping you make the moves that get you where you want to go.

Our beautiful children deserve and demand the best from us. (And I don't mean the latest Build-A-Bear or iPhone—though they adamantly attest to their need for those, too.) With good information and a bit of pluck, we can deliver the goods. And the very best of those goods are green. Yes, "green is the new black," and "long live the red, white and green!" You may have seen these catchphrases popping up in every other headline, in all sorts of media. But what does green really mean for you and your family?

Green means safe. If it's really green, it means you can finally catch a break—that you don't have to check the label (and check it twice).

Consider just a few examples:

• Wooden toys with a natural finish mean no terrifying recalls for lead-based paint.

• Organic household cleaners hold no risk of accidental poisoning.

• Some pediatricians and parents are successfully controlling ADD and ADHD without Ritalin by eliminating common food additives.

• Tomatoes grown in organic (pesticide-free) fields supply significantly higher levels of cancer-fighting antioxidants—up to ninety-seven percent higher—than conventionally grown tomatoes.

And green means safer for the world at large, too. Organic food on your dinner table protects not just your family but farmers, their workers, and wildlife, too. Not only can natural lawn care give you the luxe field of green you're pining after, but it protects your kids and pets and keeps the whole town's water supply cleaner, too.

Green is good, and it's also easy and fun. Plus, it can actually save you some greenbacks.

This is the story of our generation. We're in a new renaissance, and you and I can fund it better than the Medicis. It's time to take back our power, look great, feel great, and make a positive difference.

You're the boss of what goes in your mouth, on your body, and in your house. And being the boss has its perks—a better quality of life, for us today and our kids tomorrow. You're an integral part of Revolution Green. (Don't get nervous—I'm not asking you to take over for Castro. Revolution is quite natural. In fact, Revolution is ninety percent Evolution.)

In the U.S., we are three percent of the Earth's population but consume twenty-seven percent of the world's commercial goods.

Everything that you choose makes a difference. And it doesn't have to be ugly or crunchy, backbreaking or budget busting. Small, manageable steps can have a long and lasting impact. Especially if lots of us do them together.

It matters.

You matter.

We are history in the making. We have never had so much influence over the direction of the world. Our world.

If that all sounds a little time-consuming and lofty, I'm here to tell you it's actually incredibly doable. You're already making choices every day. Your consumer power is the path to change. And because the plethora of green claims out there can sometimes be baffling, I'll give you green guidance from the real deal, the smartest, most authoritative eco minds on the planet: my Green Gurus, experts who have devoted their energy, ingenuity, and brainpower to finding better, cleaner, greener, safer ways for the rest of us. Plus, I will share with you what I have learned (through trial and error) parenting my three great green kids.

When my first daughter was born, I founded Green Babies, an organic-cotton baby-clothing company, out of my apartment. Now, sixteen years later, hundreds of thousands of babies have worn Green Babies and we are the oldest and one of the largest organic-cotton clothing lines on the planet! I've seen the dream of organic cotton and the promise it brings for our future begin to bloom. These opportunities came about because of healthy choices I wanted to make for my child, and the support of thousands of parents who wanted to make healthy choices for their children, too.

We're in a marvelous cooperative. In this beautiful, fun, frantic life, we're all connected to one another, and I know for sure that whatever choices you make for your family affect the whole, wide world.

So come with me to a beautiful Utopia where there is enough for everyone and the future for all children is a safe haven filled with healthy food, clean air, and pure water.

Together, we can do it—and there's never been a better and more meaningful time.

Go for the Green!
—Lynda

Foreword

I'm one of the lucky ones who was brought up loving green. My father recycled, had a compost pile, planted a yearly vegetable garden, and would bring home discarded bikes that he would rehab and transform into masterpieces. There were always timers on our lights and thermostats. Even toilet water was not to be wasted—remember the saying, "If it's yellow, it's mellow. If it's brown, flush it down"? That was my dad. During the gas crunch of the seventies, he left the car parked in the driveway and bought a motorcycle to drive to work that got one hundred miles per gallon.

I fail in comparison with the tremendous example my father displayed, but I do recycle, constantly tell my kids to be conscious of their water usage, and have switched over to organic household cleaners. Unfortunately, I have only a meager herb pot, not nearly as glorious as my parents' summer vegetable garden. But I do buy organic food, give all my friends with new babies organic-cotton clothes, and love purchasing antiques and vintage clothing.

Like my father, Lynda Fassa is one of my role models when it comes to a commitment to living green. We share similar approaches to organic living, but the fact that she founded a business that benefits so many people on so many levels makes Lynda a true treasure. Not only does she use only pure, organic cotton for her clothing company, which is good for whoever wears it; she insists on it being grown under the proper conditions so that farming communities have a healthy, respectable crop and business. This helps the world on a global level.

Being a parent is the greatest joy in my life, and I want to make choices for my children that are good for them, and for the planet. I know you'll find good green guidance on everything from school lunches to nontoxic toys in Lynda's comprehensive, helpful guide *Green Kids, Sage Families.*

—Vanessa Williams

Part I 🍃

Green Acres
Is the Place
to Be

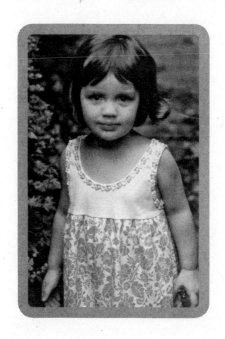

Little Sprouts Branching Out

One 🌿
Field of
Green
Dreams

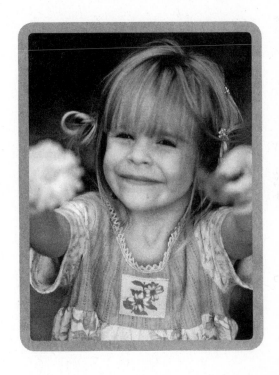

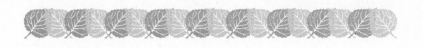

What You Need to Know to Protect Your Child from Toxins, Now That Baby's Not a Baby Anymore

I always thought a rolling lawn was a really beautiful thing. As a matter of fact, I always thought rolling along a lawn was a really beautiful thing. I guess every kid does. My sister and I grew up in the city of Chicago in the 1960s and '70s. We didn't have a backyard, but just outside our door was the beautiful and lush long length of Lincoln Park hugging Lake Michigan's turbulent shore.

A huge hit in my youth, "This land is your land, this land is my land" became my mantra—I definitely thought of the park as my land. Pulling up tufts of grass as a toddler, picnicking with my family, later enjoying surly teenage diatribes under the comforting shade of large trees. Today in the bucolic New York suburbs where I live, children spend every weekend (except the hottest summer days) kicking the soccer ball in well-cured green havens. Toddling babies still pull up tufts on the town green and sullen teens still sit under great oaks discussing parents' inequities. Generations repeat life's patterns and all seems well in my town. Growing limbs and stretching bodies should be able to enjoy the great outdoors.

But what if there was an intruder lurking, unseen in the sun and the shadows? An insidious, invisible force, intent on killing? What if it was poised under the bronze William Shakespeare statue in Lincoln Park, in your child's favorite playground, and in the cushioning of my tween's fall on the school soccer field here in the idyllic burbs?

Unfortunately, there is such an intruder. There's a killer in our midst. Pesticides and herbicides are poisons. They are designed to kill, and they do not have an off switch. What attacks stubborn weeds and pests attacks humans, as well. It's time to clean up our yards, our parks, and our plates. The next generation is counting on us.

THE BACKYARD AND BEYOND

Green Flag

Here's the good news: Ten U.S. states require or recommend the use of integrated pest management (IPM) on state-owned and state-run lands—parks, playgrounds, highways, landscapes, etc. Integrated pest management means using natural or less-toxic techniques of controlling insects wherever possible.

Red Flag

Here's the bad news: Forty states do not. That means for most of us there is no state-mandated management or control of the type and amount of pesticides and poisons used in public parks, fields, and forests. What are states doing to limit the use of toxic pesticides (which our tax dollars are funding) and the ensuing environmental and health damage they cause? Unfortunately, not very much. Why does that matter for us and our families? Because the most commonly used pesticides are neurotoxins, endocrine disrupters, and known or probable human carcinogens, and they have the greatest effect on the very young (source: Beyond Pesticides newsletter, August 2007).

According to the Centers for Disease Control, children have twice the levels of pesticides as adults. Here's what it says in their *Second National Report on Human Exposure to Environmental Chemicals*:

> Developing systems are likely to show more long-term effects of such exposure because of the added burden of growing bodies. Simply put, children's livers and kidneys do not pass out toxins as efficiently as adults do. Plus, because of the places and ways children play, they are far more likely to come into direct contact with pesticides, fertilizers and weed killers.

BEYOND RAIN MAN We don't yet know what causes autism. In the not-so-distant past it was attributed to coldhearted "refrigerator mothers." Then we moved away from that really weird idea to look for a single external cause, for example, vaccines. Right now scientists are looking at the "body burden" theory—the idea that it's a combination of multiple contributing factors including environment, genetics, and gene-environment interactions. Potential triggers being investigated include heavy metals like mercury and pesticides.

Thank goodness we are looking at what we can do to avoid this sorrow; as parents and as a society the stakes couldn't get any higher. The EPA says autism affects over one million children—that's a two hundred percent increase over the number ten years ago. 🌿

According to Beyond Pesticides, of the thirty most commonly used lawn pesticides,

nineteen are linked with cancer or carcinogenicity
thirteen with birth defects
twenty-one with reproductive effects
twenty-six with liver or kidney damage
fifteen with neurotoxicity
eleven with disruption of the endocrine (hormonal) system.

SECRET AGENT, MAN

Or maybe not such a secret. It's Agent Orange, the chemical the U.S. used in Vietnam in the 1970s to cut through some of the toughest and most tenacious tropical plants on the planet.

What does that have to do with you? One of the main ingredients of Agent Orange is 2,4-dichlorophenoxyacetic acid (2,4-D), which is still in use. In fact, it's the primary ingredient in some of the most commonly used backyard weed killers in North America.

"Why don't you kids go outside and play?" takes on new and ominous connotations if we use commercial weed killers in our yards. That means the bottles with the targeted spritzers you may have stored in your garage or on the back porch. They do seem like a great convenience. They wipe out crabgrass, dandelions, and poison ivy so quickly that they wither and die within a day or two. But as we consider how they can accomplish that, we may want to go back to a more benign approach to lawn care.

Here's what the Sierra Club of Canada has to say: "2,4-Dichloro-phenoxyacetic Acid (2,4-D) is a chlorinated phenoxy herbicide. 2,4-D has been shown to cause cellular mutations which can lead to cancer. This mutagen contains dioxins, a group of chemicals known to be hazardous to human health and to the environment."

The ingredient 2,4-D is banned for residential use in Quebec, Sweden, Denmark, and Norway, and it is highly restricted in many EU countries.

If you currently have a product containing 2,4-D and decide to toss it for your family's sake, contact your local municipality—do NOT drop it in the regular trash. It needs special handling on a "hazardous waste" pickup day. (So what were we doing spraying it in our backyard . . . ?)

Green Guru

Dr. Jane Aronson
AKA THE ORPHAN DOCTOR
PEDIATRICIAN SPECIALIZING IN INTERNATIONAL ADOPTION
FOUNDER, THE WORLDWIDE ORPHANS FOUNDATION
MOTHER

Sometimes you meet a person whose passion is so magnetic, she inspires others to action and adoration, just by the force of her being. Dr. Jane is such a person. She has committed her life to making day-to-day existence better for the children she calls "all our kids," the 150 million orphans the world over. She's a pediatrician in a highly successful private practice in Manhattan with a specialty in international adoptions. She's also a glossy-magazine favorite because of her close relationship with some of the biggest movie stars on the planet. She's a devoted mate and a busy mom. But she saw a deep need for assistance and advocacy for the kids who will be left behind, the children in foreign orphanages who will never leave for a new home. So she formed Worldwide Orphans Foundation to address the needs and improve the quality of life of orphaned kids from Ethiopia to Vietnam and everywhere in between. Check out her beautiful mission at www.wwo.org. And check out her experiences with environmental toxins, here.

"Internationally adopted children and environmental issues are forever linked, because often these kids come from developing nations where there has been a complete disrespect for the environment. And they're stuck, these communities, these countries. They have no money to solve their problems. In Ethiopia they took down all their trees to sell for lumber, because they needed the cash. But no trees mean no soil, no soil means no farming.

"In so many countries I see the destruction of children's lives by environmental devastation. I was just in Vietnam and saw hospital wards filled with kids who three generations later are suffering from the effects of Agent Orange. At the Phumey orphanage in Ho Chi Minh City, about ten percent of the one thousand children are suffering deformities and disabilities that look like they're from Agent Orange exposure; many are in a completely vegetative state. Agent Orange was applied between 1962 and 1971, but it's still having an effect. It doesn't disappear. That stuff is still in the water supply in any country where it was used.

"In contrast to Vietnam, the U.S. is a fantastically affluent society, yet we haven't protected ourselves or our children. We chopped down every forest; we relaxed environmental standards; we developed hundreds of thousands of chemicals. We have epidemic rates of ADD, ADHD, autism, and cancer.

"Every decision was based on increasing production. No one considered the side effects.

"We need to do better. We can stop damage to the environment. We can develop products that do no harm: to people, to animals, to plants. We're a world leader. We can do this, and the time is now."

THE GRASS IS ALWAYS GREENER

The pesticide label is a legally binding document. It usually comes as a little pamphlet attached to the cap or the can. Most of us just peel it off and toss it away, without realizing that that can hold the key to our pets', our kids', and our own health. Some people use pesticides and don't even know it. Next time you're in the grocery or hardware store, check out the small booklet or folded sheet attached to the container. This is the pesticide label.

You're probably using a product with chemical pesticides if you're using

- bug spray or bait

- insect repellent

- any form of a pet's flea or tick treatment or repellent, including tick collars

- hand sanitizer

- bathroom mold and mildew treatment

- kitchen disinfectants

- some swimming pool disinfectants

- most common weed killers

- certain mouthwashes and toothpastes.

PUT YOUR PESTICIDE WHERE YOUR MOUTH IS? Triclosan is a common additive to toothpastes and mouthwashes that make antigerm claims. Triclosan is classified by the FDA as a pesticide. Mmm, does your mouth feel clean now? Don't feel bad if you've fallen prey to these seductive marketing ploys. Now is our opportunity to wake up and begin to rethink product claims, and connect to our ability to make more healthful choices. 🌿

Red Flag

AS THE CLICHÉ GOES, IF IT SEEMS TOO GOOD TO BE TRUE, IT IS The next time you're reaching for an easy fix to scrubbing the bathroom, consider this: Nothing but a highly toxic herbicide (a poison designed to kill plants) can "wipe through tough mildew" in seconds. Likewise you may want to reconsider a spray that kills 99.9 percent of germs. "Kills" is the operative word here. Even hospitals are beginning to switch from powerful germicidal chemicals in all but surgical areas. Why? Because some germs are good. Also what about that 0.1 percent we didn't kill? Some scientists speculate we may be creating an army of supergerms with those that we don't wipe out with these chemical onslaughts. . . . What then?

When a product says DANGER, WARNING, or CAUTION: KEEP OUT OF REACH OF CHILDREN and you take it out to use it, just how "out of reach" is it?

Some people think they are improving their property when they have a perfect lawn. But it's not an improvement if it's laden with toxic pesticides and herbicides. My friend Tessa Hill says, "Learn to love weeds or just mow 'em down." But there are even more alternatives than that. The most effective lawn care programs begin with a clear understanding of what grass really needs in order to grow. Check out these tips from Grassroots Healthy Lawn Program (www.ghlp.org) to keep your grass truly green.

• **Feed the soil.** One of the best things you can do for your soil is to increase the soil biology by raking a half inch or so of compost into your lawn each spring and fall. If your lawn has been on a chemical diet, you may want to speed up the healing process by the addition of microbial inoculants. These "good" bacteria and fungi support beneficial microbes and earthworms. A soil test may identify the need for soil amendments, such as rock dust, kelp extract, or lime.

• **Feed the grass.** Leave grass clippings on the lawn. They provide nitrogen and reduce the amount of fertilizer needed by about one-half. (By the way, this does not contribute to thatch buildup. Thatch is an accumulation of dead, partially decomposed grass caused by excessive watering and fertilizing.) If you want to give your lawn an extra boost in the spring, choose an organic fertilizer with an NPK (nitrogen–phosphorus–potassium) ratio of approximately 3–1–2. Never use more than one pound per one thousand square feet.

• **Reseed annually.** A thick turf is one of the best ways to control weeds. Seed in late summer or early fall with a mixture of indigenous grasses, paying special attention to thin patches. Aeration of the soil will improve germination, but is not absolutely necessary unless you have compacted soil.

• **Mow high.** Set your lawn mower to the highest setting and leave it there. Grass should be between three and four inches high, allowing it to shade its roots, conserve moisture, and keep out weeds. High mowing is a better method for controlling crabgrass than herbicides. Keep blades sharp so they do not tear the grass, making it vulnerable to disease.

• **Water less, but longer.** Once-a-week watering in the early morning for several hours is the best method. Over-watering can create an ideal environment for pathogens to thrive. Take into consideration the rainfall and type of soil you have. Sandy soil needs more water than clay-based soil.

• **Control those weeds.** If you really don't like dandelions, dig them out! But you can also use an organic corn-gluten product that kills weed seeds (including crabgrass) and seedlings. It must be applied to established lawns early in the spring for several years to control problem areas. Corn gluten will also prevent grass seed from germinating, so be careful not to seed for at least two months after an application. If you hand weed large areas, fill with compost and grass seed and keep moist until grass sprouts.

• **Deal with pests naturally.** The most common pests (grubs, sod webworms, chinch bugs) can be controlled with applications of beneficial nematodes. Follow directions carefully, as they are fragile and must be kept cool and moist. Milky spore powder is an effective control for Japanese beetle grubs, and just one application can last for many years. Fungal diseases can be successfully treated with several light applications of compost or liquid-compost "tea."

Go to the Grassroots Healthy Lawn Program site at www.ghlp .org and you can even download—for free—the Green Lawn Card with easy-to-use tips for keepin' it green and healthy.

If you're lucky, you have your own little safe haven, for example, a backyard over which you have control. But if you're concerned about the persistent pesticides and other chemicals used on your parks, playgrounds, and school property—and you certainly should be—let your local, state, and federal government know that this matters to you and that you are counting on them to protect your kids. If they need some incentive, please tell them you plan on voting based on their stand on this issue. And consider supporting one of the nonprofits that will amplify your concerns and make your voice heard, such as these:

• Organic Consumers Association

• Beyond Pesticides

• Pesticide Action Network North America

• Natural Resources Defense Council

WATER, WATER EVERYWHERE, BUT NOT A DROP TO DRINK

Another reason to be concerned about pesticides is that whatever you put on your lawn is at risk of washaway from rain. That's one of the main ways dangerous chemicals get into our drinking-water supply and then into our bodies, not to mention the damage they do to water life. Atrazine is a commonly used weed killer in the U.S. (to the tune of about seventy-six billion pounds per year), even though it's been banned in many European countries. In lab tests fish and frogs exposed to atrazine begin to change their sex from male to female.

Green Guru

Janelle Hope Robbins
STAFF SCIENTIST, WATERKEEPER ALLIANCE

Janelle has a big brain, and spends most hours of her days looking for practical solutions to complex environmental problems that affect us common folks—but she also has a generous knack for explaining important things to people who might possess a little less of the gray matter than she was endowed with. Janelle is the staff scientist for Waterkeeper Alliance, a consortium of nonprofits headed by Robert F. Kennedy Jr. that works at both legal and hands-in-the-muck grassroots efforts to clean up the most precious thing on the planet, the great blue jewel—our water. Here I asked her to explain why what we put on our lawns and cars and in our bodies matters to the cleanliness, health, and safety of our most precious resource.

"Runoff or washaway is just what it sounds like: the water that runs off the ground during a storm. Runoff carries everything from your lawn or garden—poisons like pesticides and fertilizers, dog poop, soil, you name it. Big storms can make enough runoff to toss around cars and trucks like they are toys. Roofs, driveways, and sidewalks generate runoff, too. Depending on where you live, runoff may be treated before it is released to your local river, lake, or bay, but sometimes it isn't treated at all before it goes into the water. Polluted runoff is the number one source of water pollution in the United States. It causes beach closures, kills fish, and contaminates drinking water.

"It may seem like when we turn on the faucet, there is an endless stream of clear, cold, refreshing water to be had, because of the way it gushes out. But in reality, there isn't an endless supply of clean water on this Blue Planet, and in many places on earth, the water is neither clear nor safe enough to drink to be called refreshing. Drinking water typically comes from one of two main sources: wells that tap into groundwater aquifers, which are like underground lakes of water, or surface water like reservoirs, lakes, and rivers.

"Groundwater and surface water are connected by the water cycle, which is the movement of water in the environment. When it rains or snows, the water soaks into the ground to become part of an aquifer or flows into rivers, lakes, and oceans. The roots of trees and other plants draw water out of the ground. Groundwater and surface water feed each other using underground streams. The sun causes water to evaporate, forming clouds again so the cycle can continue. People are part of the water cycle, too—we are, after all, seventy percent water! We take water to drink, cook, and bathe, but it always goes back to the environment. When we flush the toilet or put water down the drain, it is treated and returned to the earth to become drinking water for someone else, somewhere else. Water is continuously recycled in the environment and the water cycle is as old as time. In fact, the water you drank today could have been dinosaur pee thousands of years ago!

"Both groundwater and surface-water sources of drinking water are recharged by precipitation and runoff. Rain and runoff can both carry contaminants, but runoff in particular can carry poisons like pesticides and heavy metals, disease-causing pathogens, and the nutrients nitrogen and phosphorus, which are responsible for the huge dead zones in the Gulf of Mexico and the Chesapeake Bay. While the U.S. has come a long way in protecting water from big polluters like factories, water is still a precious resource. Less than 0.3 percent of all the water on earth is considered to be fresh, and even less is accessible to us, so it is vital that we conserve and protect whatever water we can."

SOME WAYS TO AVOID CAUSING RUNOFF

• **Consider using native vegetation rather than a turf lawn.** Native plants are more drought- and disease-resistant and require less pesticides, fertilizer, and irrigation.

• **Use rain barrels to collect rain from gutters to water your garden and lawn, and consider planting a rain garden to soak up any extra rain or runoff from patios, sidewalks, and driveways.** This not only conserves potable water for drinking, but also reduces the amount of storm water entering our bodies of water.

• **Wash your car on your lawn instead of in the driveway.** This lets the water soak into the ground instead of running off into storm-water drains and local water bodies.

• **When walking your dog, pick up the waste and dispose of it down a toilet or throw it in a trash bin.** Never throw pet waste near storm drains, culverts, ditches, or water bodies.

• **Drain pools and spas only when test kits detect a chlorine level of zero.** Whenever possible and legal, drain pools and spas into sanitary sewers so the water can be treated.

Remember, when it comes to pesticides and herbicides, there is no us or them because (at the risk of sounding like a Zen proverb) there really is no here or there. What's used outside comes inside. We track it in on the bottoms of our shoes, or on the sleeves in which our elbows rested on the grass. Our dogs bring it home after romping in the city park, and our kids throw it on the bedroom floor where they carelessly drop their team uniforms after the game.

No one is exempt. Everyone gets exposed.

Getting that monkey off our backs will literally help you breathe easier, and may have huge implications for our children, our neighbors, and ourselves. We simply do not know who is being exposed or when "some" becomes "too much to handle." But we do know pesticides are poison. So until everyone gets on board, here's how to protect yourself and those you love.

WHAT YOU CAN DO NOW

• Immediately swear off any pesticides or weed killers on your own turf, and try to sway neighbors and friends to do the same—for their sake as well as yours. Remember, you're significantly reducing your cancer risk just by taking that one easy step.

• At your next PTA meeting, raise the question of just what is used on school property.

• Take a waterproof blanket or unzip an outdoor sleeping bag for outings on suspect greens for kids to sit and play on.

• Explain to kids of any age that pesticides are poison and any public and some private green spaces may have been sprayed. They need to take care about tasting the grass (you might be surprised, but I find this is as big a problem with tweens and teens as toddlers).

• Make sure kids know to stay away from pesticides. Those little yellow warning flags must be put in the ground—by law—to alert you when a toxic pesticide has recently been applied. Teach your children what the flags mean: STAY AWAY. (Too bad the squirrels and birds can't read. . . .)

• Have kids take showers immediately after playing on school or town fields. (Added benefit—they'll smell better at the family dinner table, too!)

• Go on record with your community and school system in favor of integrated pest management. Bring them some terrific real-world science info you download from www .beyondpesticides.org and you may make some converts.

IN THE GARDEN, AS IN LIFE, ALL THINGS GROW WITH LOVE

OK, after all that doom and gloom, here comes the fun part. Time to create your own little piece of paradise.

Before we moved to the bucolic burbs, when we lived in Manhattan, I always had my kids by the hand or buckled tight in their strollers when we were outside. I used to fantasize about us all lying on our backs in the evening looking up at the changing sky and counting stars. Those dreams instantly came true when we left the city behind. We bought our ramshackle house for two reasons: (1) we could afford it, and (2) it had a terrific, large, sloping backyard.

Our evenings were filled with natural adventures. We'd speed through homework to run outside at twilight with Ball jars to catch and release fireflies. I was terribly lazy about mowing the lawn, so it looked something like the Illinois prairie. True, this meant we needed to be especially vigilant checking the kids and dog for ticks (Lyme, Connecticut, for which Lyme disease is named, is not far away), but besides possibly harboring less-than-welcome guests (as any natural space can), my yard was, and is, a safe haven for a biodiverse group of beneficial insects, fascinating and adorable wild animals—and my growing gremlins, too.

VICTORY IS MINE!

We were so enthralled with our green space that we planted and carefully tended our own victory garden. (Brief lesson for those of you who, like me, snoozed through your tenth-grade U.S. history class: During World War II Americans were asked to help grow their own food in so-called Victory Gardens in their own backyards so more agricultural and manufacturing power could be directed to the war effort.)

Our six-by-eight-foot victory garden was such a huge success that my husband used to go out and survey it every morning with his hands on his hips and a look of satisfaction, as if he

were a wealthy European land baron. We had so many tomatoes we invited all the neighborhood kids and had a pickin'
party. There really is no better way to connect your kids (and
yourself) to the drama of our interdependence on one another,
the big circle of life, than to plant something and watch it grow.
Did I say drama? Well, there's a lot of comedy out there, too. . . .

EAT LIKE A LADY

One summer we were visited by little green bugs that I originally
thought were adorable, but soon discovered were voracious aphids.
Little clouds of light green would descend upon my English rose-
bushes and chow down until there was not much left. It was almost biblical. I'd heard you could order ladybugs and they would
clean up the problem, so off to the Internet I went and in a few
days they arrived, sleepy but safe, in a beautiful sisal bag. I'll tell
you, when we let 'em out, my kids were so enchanted you'd have
thought I'd ordered thousands of pixies and leprechauns. And
the problem was solved within the week.

Our backyard adventures really are some of the happiest and
most lasting memories I have of my young children. There is a
tremendous amount of joy and fulfillment to be gained from a
little time in the garden.

Come meet someone who may take you down the garden
path, too.

She's a Green Guru who has made a lifetime out of giving kids
the gift of gardening.

Green Guru

Joyce Walsack

FOUNDER, GARDEN TYKES, ONLINE PURVEYOR OF
NATURAL-GARDENING SUPPLIES FOR KIDS
MOM AND GRANDMOTHER

I grew up in an urban environment, where gardening wasn't a day-to-day or even a month-to-month part of my childhood. Lucky for me, though, memories of my favorite grandmother's house (appropriately her name was Rozi) and her glorious flower-filled backyard are part of my psychic heritage. Bumblebees and butterflies, prized zinnias, and fragrant roses are stored in my memories like heirlooms.

I believe that any kind of natural gardening is meaningful and conducive to all kinds of positive organic growth for children. I am especially happy because I found someone (a grandmother!) who can help make all those beautiful things possible for you and your kids, whatever your geographic or demographic profile.

"I've run the gamut—my kids are in their thirties and my grandson, Sam, is four and granddaughter, Susanna, is two—and I understand what kids of all ages need to love gardening.

"Basically, the garden needs to be relaxed. Let the kids make their own little trench, even if it's not straight. If they don't put the seeds in exactly eighteen inches apart, it doesn't matter. Nature is very forgiving. The important thing is just to be together outdoors.

"What attracted me to the whole idea of family gardening is that, without a lot of preaching and without a lot of talking, you can pass something valuable on to the next generation.

"One day I was teaching my nieces, aged three and five, how to cut zinnias—how to find just the right spot so you don't cut the buds that haven't flowered yet, in order to preserve the next life. Even as I was talking, I thought, 'Why am I bothering? Are they really going to get it?' Then I saw the older one showing her sister just the right way, and I realized this is time so well spent. Even if they don't remember the specifics, so what? You're cultivating a love of nature, of something without TV, computers, or sound effects.

"Nature is amazing. It speaks to something deep inside of us. You don't need an acre, just a little corner and a few minutes."

GARDEN TIPS FOR EVERYONE, FROM LITTLE TYKES TO TWEENS

Gardening with children is just like gardening with adults in the sense that it can be as simple or as elaborate as you choose. The act of scattering some seeds and waiting for Mother Nature to take care of the rest is all that's required to make you a "gardener." As adult facilitators we should be planting ideas along with the seeds.

In chronological order and labeled by age, here are some

wonderful ideas from Joyce on what can happen when you take children into the garden.

All Ages

Create a Garden Journal

Create a scrapbook/journal that ties all your gardening activities together. Every age group can contribute. Older children might create weather reports, rain measurements, and planting and harvesting statistics; younger ones can contribute crayon drawings, seed samples, dried leaves and petals. Pages can include Planting Day, Weeding Day, Picking Day, and, our favorite, a Superlatives Page documenting the heaviest tomato, longest cucumber, or most impressive pumpkin.

Ages Two to Five

Plant the Seeds!

Sowing seeds is a good project for the littlest ones. To make it more of an activity, start by sharing a garden-themed storybook. Two excellent ones for this age group are *Pumpkin Pumpkin* by Jeanne Titherington and Ruth Krauss' classic *The Carrot Seed.*

Even the youngest child can plant seeds. For plants with large seeds, like beans, peas, pumpkins, and watermelons, use a dowel, a wooden spoon, or some other tool to make holes the correct depth and distance apart. Then let the little one drop the seeds in and cover the hole, patting the soil by hand. For very small seeds such as carrots, make a furrow the correct depth. Prepare a mixture combining sand or very fine soil with the seeds and let the children sprinkle it into the prepared furrow. Be sure to water gently, obviously a great job for these youngest gardeners. While a kid-sized watering can is perfect for this job, it isn't necessary. Many items in your recycling container can easily be made into safe, effective watering devices.

Ages Five to Eight

Choose Your Crops

Collaborate with your children on a "wish list" of flowers and vegetables you would like to grow. Tour the grocery store or farmers' market and take suggestions while discussing the origins of various items and their suitability for planting in your area. Ask them, "Can we grow oranges in Vermont?" and "Do beans grow in trees or on bushes?" For some children this may be the first they've thought about the origins of the food they are served in your home. Let them record the choices made during these trips. Seed catalogs make another great source of ideas for your garden plan.

Ages Eight to Twelve

Lay Out the Garden and Schedule the Planting

Have the gardeners measure your available garden space and plot the layout on graph paper. Discuss how to choose the proper scale for your drawing. Consult planting directions for each type of seed or plant and calculate the distance between rows and plants. Determine the average date of last frost in your area, and using a calendar and your seed-package instructions, decide when to plant each crop. Assist with planning successive plantings for a longer harvest. Equip your gardeners with a tape measure or yardstick, some stakes, and some colorful yarn or twine to mark off the rows.

BUTTERFLIES ARE FREE (OR ALMOST)

Purchase a good-quality organic butterfly mix. Butterfly seeds are made up of many varieties of plants known to attract butterflies. Depending on your location, some will do better than others and some may not grow at all. That's the beauty of a wildflower mix—you never know exactly what to expect. Choose a sunny spot with good drainage, and plant in spring or fall.

Start by putting the seeds in the freezer for two days; then take them out for one day. Repeat three or four times to give your seeds a really good start. Then plant, in full sun, one-eighth to one-fourth inch deep. Be sure to water and weed your butterfly garden when it is starting out. (Careful, though—in the beginning it can be hard to tell the weeds from the flowers!)

Keep your seeds and seedlings well watered. One day they will be strong and drought-resistant, but in the beginning they need extra care.

While you wait for your garden to bloom, check out your local library to read up on butterflies. You want to be able to identify them when they flock to your beautiful garden! There are books available for any age level.

Green Guru

Eric Vinje
FOUNDER, PLANET NATURAL

Don't have a backyard to explore the wild in? Meet Green Guru Eric Vinje, founder of Planet Natural, a mail-order catalog and Web site (www.planetnatural.com) specializing in organic- and

indoor-gardening supplies. An avid gardener, he has been growing organically with his family in Bozeman, Montana, for more
than twenty years. (Hint: He's The Man if you need ladybugs to
deal with an outdoor aphid problem like I had!)

"Gardening indoors is a great option for families without a
lot of outdoor space, or those living in climates with cold
winters. While almost anything can be grown indoors in
containers, certain herbs and vegetables are especially appropriate. Basil, cilantro, oregano, dill, and thyme are but a
few of the herbs that take as well to containers as they do to
spicing up dinner. Vegetables like beans, lettuce, tomatoes,
and radishes also grow easily inside.

"To get the whole family involved, take a field trip to the
local nursery to pick out seeds or starter plants. Children
will feel more invested in the project if they get to pick
what they grow. You'll also need containers, an organic
potting mix (garden soil doesn't work well in containers),
grow lights (if you don't get strong sunlight in your house),
and an organic liquid fertilizer (or you can make your own
compost tea).

"Fill the containers about halfway with the potting mix,
set the plants in, and then fill the rest, leaving an inch or
two at the top of the pot for watering. Water daily, or however often is needed to keep the soil as moist as a wrung-out
sponge. You'll need to add an organic liquid fertilizer every
week or so, since watering leaches nutrients from the soil.
Then, wait for yummy organic herbs and vegetables to ap-
pear!"

INDOOR GARDENING ESSENTIALS

• Container. Buy containers at a nursery, discount store, or thrift shop, or make your own. Almost anything can be turned into a gardening container (old pots, buckets, kids' dump trucks); just drill a few holes in the bottom for drainage and set it on a plate to catch the water that seeps out.

• Potting soil. Buy an organic potting mix from a nursery or online.

• Grow lights. Ask at a nursery or order online from a company like Planet Natural.

• Seeds or starter plants. Both can be purchased at a nursery. Seeds can be ordered online or from catalogs.

• Organic liquid fertilizer. Purchase at a nursery, order online, or make your own compost tea.

HOW TO MAKE COMPOST TEA

1. Fill a bucket about one-third full with finished compost.

2. Add water until the bucket is full.

3. Let the bucket sit for at least a few hours, or up to three or four days.

4. Using cheesecloth or a fine screen, strain the mixture into another container. (Anything left over can be thrown into the garden or back into the compost bin.)

5. Add water to the liquid until it is the color of weak tea.

6. Apply the compost tea to the soil around your plants.

GREEN AT A GLANCE

 Evergreen: Invest in a truly green yard and swear off synthetic pesticides, herbicides, and fertilizers, whether you do it yourself or hire out lawn care.

Pea green: Make your own little Green Haven with an organic garden, and involve the kids!

Spring green: Limit your kids' skin-to-grass contact when you are not sure of what's been used, and insist on showers and baths after outdoor time in these spaces.

Two 🌿

Garden
of Eatin'

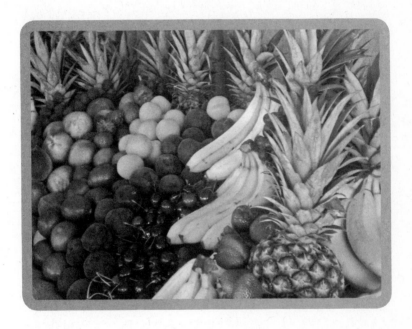

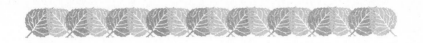

How to Get the Most from What Goes in Your Family's Mouths

My super-gorgeous sister, Dawn, always says a bad food addiction is harder to overcome than any other dependency. Her theory is (1) everyone can see your problem, clear as day (or tight as my jeans), and (2) you need to eat every single day for the rest of your life. So unlike with alcohol, cigarettes, or drugs, you'll constantly have to face the object of your (sometimes) unhealthy or overzealous desire. It can't ever be avoided or shut out completely.

On the other hand, of course, food is a really wonderful thing, a gift from the planet to your palate. Food picks you up, keeps you going, and hopefully tastes terrific to boot. Plus it's a great way to strengthen family bonds.

Having grown up in the 1970s, I practically turn into one of Pavlov's dogs when I hear the crinkle of cellophane. I never met a bag of Fritos I didn't like. My friend Alice Gee, who was a roommate of mine when we were both literally starving models in Milan, loved to say, "Food is only a happy means of transportation for salt." Well, Alice doesn't live here anymore, and I've got news for you—it's also a means of transportation for fat and sugar. Yum! And I'm not the only one who loves this junk. Most American kids are chomping convenience and snack foods by the fistful. And as bad a rap as salt, fat, and sugar have, there are some things you may want to be even more concerned about.

Just what is passing into our grocery carts under the guise of food? There's a lot more than calories, carbs, and protein in them thar vittles.

THE SWEET LIFE

Pop quiz #1: What smells like vanilla, tastes like vanilla (sort of), and is spelled in a confusingly similar way to vanilla?

Answer: Vanillin.

The difference between vanilla and vanillin is more than the letters *i* and *n*.

For one thing, the word with fewer letters will probably cost you a few bucks more, but in this case less is more—in many ways. Vanillin, which is widely used to inexpensively replace its natural counterpart—vanilla—is actually a synthetically derived flavoring made from the waste of wood pulp! Toxicology reports conclude vanillin is "harmful if swallowed," yet the FDA approved it as a food additive. I'm sorry, what part of "eating" does the FDA not understand? Apparently the part where we swallow the food!

They said they approved vanillin because, as a flavoring, it'd be used in small quantities. Sorry, but since the original, vanilla, is NOT harmful if swallowed, why don't we just stick with that?

Be careful out there—if you're looking to avoid vanillin, it's not enough just to double-check the brown bottles in the spice section of the supermarket. Vanillin is so cheap, it substitutes for the real thing just about everywhere, especially in cakes, cookies, and candies, even very pricey ones. So get out your grandma bifocals and read the fine print to see where vanillin lurks.

Check out some of the science stats at www.physchem.ox.ac .uk/MSDS/VA/vanillin.html.

Green Flag
Got a sweet tooth but lookin' for the real thing?

Here's the crème de la crème in terms of chocolates:

- Theo

- Whole Foods 365 Organic Everyday Value chocolate bar

- Endangered Species organic chocolate (www.chocolatebar .com, where your purchase also helps support endangered animals)

- Newman's Own

- Dagoba

Even Hershey's now has organic chocolate with only natural ingredients!

BLACK GOLD, TEXAS TEA
Pop quiz #2: How many cherries are in cherry Jell-O?

Yup, none.

OK, that one was pretty easy. But do you know what Yellow No. 7 is made from? Or Red No. 3? They are petroleum derivatives. Yes, that's just what it sounds like. Most synthetic colors you'll see listed on food labels as FD&C (Food, Drug, and Cosmetics) are made from petroleum (they used to be made from coal tar, yum). Put that in your car and drive it, Uncle Jed. Just don't put it in my kids' candy, please!

And in case you think the FDA is on top of protecting you, consider this: Way back in 1982 Ellen Silbergeld, chief toxicologist for the Environmental Defense Fund, discovered a relationship between Red Dye No. 3 and hyperactivity in genetically susceptible children. According to a *New York Times* story of that same year:

> Miss Silbergeld, who was formerly a researcher with the National Institute of Neurological Diseases, discovered that Red No. 3 (which is being used in place of Red No. 2, a known carcinogen, and Red No. 40, a suspected carcinogen) interferes with certain forms of metabolism. Miss Silbergeld said that just a small proportion of children may react adversely to the dye. "However," she added, "the reaction is genetically linked and appears to confirm the neurotoxicity of Red No. 3."

Consider this (*warning: gross info to follow*). Red Dye No. 3, which causes thyroid cancer in animals, is also used as a pesticide to kill flies' eggs (maggots) in manure piles (source: U.S. Environmental Protection Agency).

And if you're not running for the bathroom from that, consider this less-sickening but equally baffling fact: Red No. 3 is considered so suspect, it is not allowed to color the wax on cheese. Yet it *is* allowed (and oft used) as a color in candy! Hmm, the outside of cheese that you peel and throw away . . . or candy, which you eat . . . ?

To boot, recent studies show these artificial colors are potentially affecting all our kids with the chemical version of ants-in-their-pants.

In a groundbreaking 2007 study published in *The Lancet* (the UK's equivalent of our *New England Journal of Medicine*), it's been determined that "normal" kids exhibit ADD- and ADHD-type symptoms after ingesting relatively small amounts of common food additives, specifically food colored and preserved with synthetic ingredients.

As described in a September 6, 2007, *Time* magazine story entitled "Hyper Kids? Cut Out Preservatives," the *Lancet* study showed that what many of us give our kids in the form of a school snack or an after-soccer pick-me-up may in fact be a chemical-laden bomb, going off in ways that are unpredictable, uncontrollable, and certainly unwanted.

The *Time* story reported:

> A carefully designed study published in the British journal *The Lancet* shows that a variety of common food dyes and the preservative sodium benzoate—an ingredient in many soft drinks, fruit juices and salad dressings—do cause some kids to become measurably more hyperactive and distractible.

The study looked at three hundred kids, each of whom was given a fruit drink once per day. The drinks were either (1) a typical juice drink with sodium benzoate and synthetic color, (2) one with lesser amounts than the average of each of the above, or (3) a totally natural fruit drink.

For three weeks the kids were independently evaluated by observers who did not know which drink a child was getting. The results? Many kids—none of whom had ever exhibited hyperactivity prior to taking part in the study—became noticeably hyperactive after drinking the beverage with higher levels of additives.

The *Time* story goes on to say, "The [*Lancet*] paper warns that 'these adverse effects could affect the child's ability to benefit from the experience of school.' "

TASTE THE RAINBOW

I love candy. I don't mean the classy Godiva kind, either. Toss me some Hot Tamales and I can handle the ensuing visit to the dentist. Favorites like Starburst feel like true love (oh, succulent Starburst, parting is such sweet sorrow—but part from my adored I must, because Starburst is not vegetarian). And for years I considered fruit roll-ups to be the equivalent of a serving of fruit for either me or my kids. But in all of the above, there's something troubling lurking beneath those fabu, eye-entrancing colors. Even as they mimic the best of nature (buttercups, monarch butterflies, Ceylon rubies, a coveted electric blue Corvette . . . whoops, I guess that's not natural), they mock the divine makeup of those palettes. Those colors were concocted in the lab, and they are not without documented side effects.

Look at what the Center for Science in the Public Interest (www.cspinet.org) has to say about artificial colorings:

Most artificial colorings are synthetic chemicals that do not occur in nature. The use of coloring usually indicates that fruit or another natural ingredient has not been used.

• **Blue No. 2 (Pet Food, Beverages, Candy).** The largest study suggested, but did not prove, that this dye caused brain tumors in male mice. The FDA concluded that there is "reasonable certainty of no harm."

• **Red No. 3 (Cherries in Fruit Cocktail, Candy, Baked Goods).** The evidence that this dye caused thyroid tumors in rats is "convincing," according to a 1983 review committee report requested by the FDA. The FDA's recommendation that the dye be banned was overruled by pressure from elsewhere in the Reagan administration.

• **Yellow No. 6 (Beverages, Sausage, Baked Goods, Candy, Gelatin).** Industry-sponsored animal tests indicated that this dye, the third-most widely used, causes tumors of the adrenal gland and kidney. In addition, small amounts of several carcinogens contaminate Yellow No. 6. However, the FDA reviewed those data and found reasons to conclude that Yellow No. 6 does not pose a significant cancer risk to humans. Yellow No. 6 may cause occasional allergic reactions. (Source: www.CSPInet.org.)

Green Guru

Jane Hersey
DIRECTOR, THE FEINGOLD ASSOCIATION
AUTHOR
MOM

I'd heard about the Feingold method of helping kids with learning disabilities, ADD, ADHD, and autism, but, I admit, until recently I didn't really pay it any attention (maybe it was that box of Hot Tamales?). My kids have no problems with academics (knock wood), so beyond the ordinary lack of attention to, say, me asking them to set the table for dinner, I did not have the focusing issues that parents whose kids are struggling in school do. Basically, I didn't "get it," the food/ Feingold thing. But a much-needed closer look told me loud and clear that for kids with any stimuli sensitivities, what they eat can make the difference between functioning well and a truly bad day. Thousands of parents who face daunting problems with the kids they love, problems ranging from irritable outbursts to repetitive behaviors including head banging, have found relief by following the Feingold system. In 1973, Dr. Benjamin Feingold, a pediatric allergist from California, proposed that salicylates, artificial colors, and artificial flavors caused hyperactivity (what we now call ADHD) in children. Many parents who follow his recommendations to eliminate them from their kids' diets say their kids experience tremendous relief from the symptoms that plagued them.

Meet Green Guru Jane Hersey, director of the Feingold Association, and author of *Why Can't My Child Behave?*

"A specialized form of EEG enabling researchers to map the brain's electrical activity has provided objective proof that some children diagnosed with an attention disorder do not have any disorder at all. They are simply reacting to a food or a food additive. Certain foods may not only influence clinical symptoms but may also alter brain electrical activity. These tests now map out what we suspected but couldn't see before: that what you put in your mouth affects behavior.

"If you take your dog to the vet because he is acting strange, the vet always asks what your dog ate. If you take your child to the doctor because of behavioral difficulties, he never asks what your child ate. That just doesn't make any sense! If we don't think food affects us, why do we try to eat in a healthy way? Why do so many people take vitamins? For food-sensitive individuals, synthetic additives and/or salicylates may be a factor in antisocial traits, compulsive aggression, self-mutilation, difficulty in reasoning, stuttering, and a host of other effects. Thousands of parents of these affected kids have had tremendous relief by following simple guidelines for diet, notably by eliminating certain food additives like synthetic colors and certain preservatives such as Red No. 3 and BHT.

Feingold counts two hundred thousand active members. Imagine the impact on the families of those kids going from dysfunctional to functional because of what they eat. Then you can begin to understand the significance of the Feingold Association motto: Good food makes for good lives.

Check out the hundreds of letters from Feingold users on their site, www.feingold.org. Here's a peek at a few:

"We took my son off food with BHT and now his asthma is completely gone."

"I don't know how we managed before."

"You have kept me out of the hospital."

"Now her teacher says she is just like all the other kids."

"Her doctors are astonished."

IT'S NOT NICE TO FOOL MOTHER NATURE

Until recently much of the established medical community considered the Feingold "treat with food" approach total bunk.

But common sense tells us that what our kids eat quite naturally (or *un*naturally) affects how they act. After all, it is the food they eat that is building their bodies. Now science agrees.

Meanwhile, there is still more to be concerned about that's not even listed on the ingredient pane.

WHEN THE SNACK ATTACKS

In the first week of September my usual twenty-minute grocery-shopping trip morphs into a grueling two-hour quest for the holy grail: the-healthy-snack-that-my-kids-will-actually-consume-when-at-school (insert angelic music here).

On one such recent sojourn I happened upon what looked like pure gold: Baked Naturals Pretzel Thins from Pepperidge Farm. The low-gloss box (made of recycled cardboard) appealed to my "natural" instincts, as did the vividly printed proclamation "Natural, No Preservatives." But perhaps most attractive of all were the words "savory cheddar, baked with real cheddar cheese."

My eleven-year-old, Mina, loves a savory snack (just like her mama) and she be lovin' cheese. However, she's one of the estimated thirty percent of Americans who are MSG (monosodium glutamate) sensitive. Reactions range from dizziness to fainting to depression, a condition you may have heard called "Chinese Restaurant Syndrome." Mina gets really cranky and sometimes even develops a migraine headache if she eats anything flavored with MSG. So, of course, I'm a careful label reader—no MSG for my kid.

MSG is a powerful flavor enhancer, and very cheap, to boot. So it makes sense for companies to add it to, well, almost everything, because MSG makes even low-grade food taste terrific. Ever wonder why after you've eaten "barbecue flavor" chips, the regular chips just won't cut it? Or why, once you've cracked open a bag of Doritos, you often finish the whole thing in just one sitting, regardless of the size of the bag? MSG isn't called an excitotoxin for nothing.

When I was growing up, MSG wasn't just for processed foods. It was heavily advertised on TV under the brand name Accent with a jaunty jingle that went, "A little Accent, like a little love, food needs Accent!" (That still rolls around in my head along with other memorable taglines like "I can't believe I ate the whole thing" and the great Orson Welles saying, "We will sell no wine before its time." Oh yes, and "A mind is a terrible thing to waste," although, apparently, I did waste mine with too much TV watching. . . .) Accent is still in existence, but its ads seem to have faded to black, perhaps because the public perception of MSG became so negative.

But I digress. Back to Mina's snack.

I confidently dove right in and bought the Baked Naturals Pretzel Thins. I tried them out on Mina later that day (I thought it better to see if she liked them before I loaded them into her schoolbag the following week) and yes, she did like them. In fact, she *loved* them. I thought I had found the answer to my kid's snack needs. But very quickly, the happy bubble burst. Within ten minutes she was bouncing off the walls; another ten and she was screaming at her sister to shut up; ten more still and she was in bed with a raging headache and the curtains drawn.

I called the company. After listening to a folksy recording assuring me they were so durn happy to receive my call, and something to the effect of "It sure as heck won't take long before we'll be on the line," I'll be doggone if they weren't right—sure 'nough, a human (albeit a much less folksy one) came on to hear my plea. "My daughter is highly MSG sensitive," I said, "and she is suffering symptoms similar to those I know to be MSG related after eating your pretzels, but I can't see MSG listed anywhere on the label." The response? "Pepperidge Farm does not manufacture any flavorings with monosodium glutamate."

Oh, what carefully chosen words!

Amazing as it may sound, in the U.S., a company is allowed to sell food products that include MSG, a substance that a large percentage of the population is sensitive to, and not name the ingredient on the label. This is a weird and tricky loophole that works like this: If the company does not manufacture the actual ingredient, but buys it to use in the final product, they do not need to disclose exactly what it's made of. Such ingredients are often hidden behind the term "natural flavorings" (yes, MSG is natural—sort of) or "smoke flavoring" or "hydrolyzed corn, soy, or vegetable flavoring." They can further refuse even to acknowledge the ingredients when asked (as in my case) by claiming the makeup of the flavorings are "company secrets."

Shame on those companies!

Can you imagine the number of concerned and confused parents? (Maybe you're one of them.) MSG is widely considered a trigger for behavioral outbursts in kids who suffer from ADD or ADHD. How many extra doses of Ritalin are doled out because of reactions to hidden MSG? How many squirming little tushies can't stay in their seats after snack time at school?

Our kids have been wronged here, and we parents have, amazingly, and perhaps even deliberately, been kept in the dark.

To find out more and check out a vast litany of potential reactions to MSG, go to the heartfelt and hugely comprehensive www.msgmyth.com.

Also, the nonprofit Truth in Labeling has a great list of tricky names manufacturers use to hide the MSG in their labels (www.truthinlabeling.org).

KNOWING WHERE TO LOOK

According to an article in *Experience Life* magazine (March–April 2003), here's a quick list of potentially suspect ingredients to watch for (when in doubt, call the manufacturer to inquire).

• Ingredients that may contain thirty to sixty percent MSG: hydrolyzed vegetable protein, hydrolyzed protein, hydrolyzed plant protein, plant protein extract, sodium caseinate, calcium caseinate, yeast extract, textured protein, autolyzed yeast, hydrolyzed oat flour, Accent.

• Ingredients that may contain twelve to forty percent MSG: malt extract, malt flavoring, bouillon, broth, stock, natural flavoring, natural beef or chicken flavoring, seasoning, spices

• Ingredients that may contain some MSG: carrageenan, enzymes, soy protein concentrate, soy protein isolate, whey protein concentrate, some soy milk

Sources: FDA backgrounder #BG-95-16 (available at www.cfsan.fda.gov/~lrd/msg.html) and *In Bad Taste: The MSG Syndrome*, by George R. Schwartz, MD.

Reading the Fine Print

MSG isn't the only three-letter word—uh, three-letter ingredient thing—that may be causing behavioral problems in our kids. Watch out for these, too:

- **Butylated Hydroxytoluene (BHT)** (Cereals, Chewing Gum, Potato Chips, Oils, Etc.)

BHT is used to keep oils and fats from going "bad." But in some animal studies it increased the risk of cancer. It's also been proven to be stored in human fat.

- **Butylated Hydroxyanisole (BHA)** (Cereals, Chewing Gum, Potato Chips, Vegetable Oil)

BHA is another substance used to extend the shelf life of fats and oils used as ingredients in other foods. It's also been shown in some animal studies to cause cancer. The U.S. Department of Health and Human Services considers BHA to be "reasonably anticipated to be a human carcinogen." However, the Food and Drug Administration still permits BHA to be used in foods.

THE FAMILY PLAN: THE UNBEARABLE HEAVINESS OF BEING

Here's what we know: We're a nation in crisis, a big fat crisis, and it's related to the food we eat and how we eat it. For the first time in our history, studies estimate our children will not live as long as we do. One of the main reasons is poor diet. We eat food that lacks nutrients, and we eat too much. But what should we do? There is a plethora of "answers" out there, from South Beach to fruit flush—but what can we realistically do when we have a family to feed?

First, let's look at where we are:

- Nearly one in three children ages six to nineteen is overweight or at risk of becoming overweight. The same is true for one in five toddlers and preschoolers (ages two to five). This has doubled in the past twenty years.

- For older children and adolescents (ages nine to eighteen), eating as a family improves consumption of fruits, vegetables, grains, fiber, vitamins, calcium, and other minerals.

- Young people (ages nine to fourteen) who have more frequent family dinners eat less fried food and saturated fats and drink less soda than those who do not eat together as a family.

GOOD TIMES AT THE KITCHEN TABLE

Want to take back your power, preserve your loved ones' health, and add some quality family time (and cheap entertainment to boot)? Here are some fun and unconventional ideas to turn ordinary dinner into family-fun night. Plus it takes into account what for many of us is the biggest hurdle—how everyone can have it their way!

If your family is not used to having many meals together, you might want to consider trying to work it in one night at a time. Pick one evening a week for a family dinner. Choose a menu that's easily pleasing for everyone, and make participation *en famille* mandatory. (Extra note to parents of tweens and teens: In the beginning they may moan and groan, but within a couple of weeks they are looking forward to it.)

WEEKLY FAMILY DINNER NIGHT (LAUGHS AND STORIES OPTIONAL)

Easy as Pie

In the refrigerated-food section of most supermarkets you can pick up ready-to-spread-and-bake pizza dough—this is the basis for a foolproof family dinner. In addition to the dough, all you'll need is natural, preferably organic, red tomato pasta sauce (Newman's Own and Ragú are both great); shredded mozzarella cheese (Organic Valley's is, you guessed it, organic, and pretty widely available); and whatever toppings your family likes: olives, mushrooms, fresh tomatoes—let the imagination rule!

Get the family in the kitchen (ask 'em to wash up first) and lay out two or three cookie sheets. After you have had the dough rise (much easier than it sounds—follow directions on package), simply divide the dough balls into equal portions for everyone and lay out your topping ingredients on the kitchen countertop or table, like a salad bar. Let everybody pull and stretch their own dough and make their own personal pizza. Pop their creations in the oven and in about twenty minutes, voilà, fun family pizza dinner—and no fights over the toppings!

Pasta Bar

Same idea, but waaaayyyy easier. Get sixteen ounces of whatever-kind-you-like pasta. Cook and drain.

Set it on the table and provide grated Parmesan, olives, fresh tomatoes, bocconcini (little balls of fresh mozzarella), spices like garlic, oregano, and red pepper, packaged pesto, and jarred red sauce.

We do this twice a week and it is a super-economical, ultra-entertaining dinner. When I feel like we're missing greens, I toss some fresh spinach in with the cooked pasta and it steams itself on contact—the added vitamin quotient is huge!

Opposite-Day Breakfast for Dinner

Omelets, hash browns, pancakes, French toast, or scrambled eggs (egg whites if you're watching your cholesterol) are a very satisfying meal center. And little kids adore "opposite day" breakfast for dinner (sorry, Cap'n Crunch doesn't count).

Why not omelets or French toast? Honestly they're very economical, plus a crowd-pleaser. And did you know that real maple syrup has tons of minerals, so it's sweetly satisfying but also surprisingly wholesome? Don't let the price give you sticker shock. You need to use way less than supermarket "pancake syrup" for the great effect. Plus it's the ultimate in terms of sustainable farming.

The adults might do the cooking, but kids LOVE to break eggs (try to be forgiving as you crunch a little shell). Any involvement is fun and empowering for the young folks, and will equip them with responsibility for not only what goes in their mouths but maybe what goes in the cart, too, when you're shopping together.

Say Cheese and Thank You

Well, by now you probably get that none of my family members like to eat the exact same thing. However, we do like to connect at the table. So here's another easy-on-the-pocketbook but rich-in-healthful-nutrients meal that can be customized for individual tastes.

I like to use wraps, but you can just as easily opt for whole wheat toast. Lay out your ingredients smorgasbord-style, starting with the wrap/toast and a selection of condiments such as mustard, mayonnaise (sparingly), olive paste, or pesto. Next put out two or three kinds of sliced cheese, followed by sliced veggies and shredded greens. Even young kids can help wash and shred the greens.

Again, everyone gets what they like, but you all get to sit down together. Leftovers can be school lunches the next day.

Lettuce Entertain You:
Hummus, Lettuce, and Tomato Sandwiches

If you haven't tried the Middle Eastern favorite hummus, you're in for a savory treat. "A delicious taste sensation," my little Nadia used to say to her apprehensive friends.

You can make your own if you have a good food processor. You'll need

2 cans garbanzo beans, drained and rinsed
4 tablespoons pure tahini
½ cup olive oil
juice of 3 lemons
4 cloves garlic, crushed in salt
1 teaspoon cumin

Just blend it all together and you will be delighted with this savory, protein-rich spread!

Serve with pita or make HLTs: BLTs minus the bacon but with the hummus—sounds different, but the salty, strong flavor has the same satisfying effect—and almost zero carbon issues!

▶ This one's fun because there's a job for everyone in the prep, but if you're really in a hurry, there are some great ready-made brands of hummus. My favorite, Tribe, is preservative free and even comes in different flavored varieties.

Eat Your Wedgies (No, Not That Kind
of Wedgie—Ewww)

This is fun! Get the longest baguette or Italian bread you can find (if you've got a big family or big appetites, you may need two). These are available, and usually fresh daily, at any major grocery store. When choosing the bread, look for one that says "all-natural" and "no preservatives." Avoid the words

"dough conditioner"

"BHT"

"artificial flavoring."

Lay out whatever you love for the wedges, let older kids cut off and halve a chunk (you do that for little ones, of course), and let 'em pile it high.

Consider serving a side of soup. If you have a food processor, a creamy veggie soup is usually as easy as one (steam), two (add milk or cream), three (puree). If you're too swamped, pick up a ready-made soup. Remember though, many store-bought soups contain weird preservatives. Read the label carefully (as a general rule, the kind in a rectangular paper carton is more natural than its canned cousins).

I can pretty much guarantee you will have a joyous, connected time with your family if you try this once or twice a week for a month. When that takes hold, consider working in another night a week until, ideally, eating together becomes something of the norm. It is such a simple yet powerful way of connecting with family. (Remember: The first couple of tries can be fraught with some irritability and quarreling, but these simmer right down in a week or two.) The apple of my eye, my firstborn (now fifteen), groans about the obligation of coming home early or leaving her room for these get-togethers, but she clearly enjoys them, and occasionally even cracks a smile between bites.

Final thoughts: I know a few of these suggestions are cold plates, but what's more important, hot food or actually eating together and having everyone reasonably happy? Families are just so busy that trying to prep, cook, and serve a hot meal and also expecting everyone to sit their tushes at the table at the same time can set us up for family-dinner failure.

Whatever you have for dinner, as long as you have it together, give yourself a hand (of applause) and ask for a hand (of help). Most of all, cut yourself some slack—remember, Mother knows best, and what she really knows is, no one has fun if it's stressful.

MEAT THE PARENTS: WHY VEGGIES MAKE SO MUCH SENSE

My kids have never eaten meat or chicken. In the town where we live, they are the only vegetarians in a school system of twenty-five hundred children. (Oh, wait, that's not actually true. There are two other children, from a family of devout Hindus. A school nurse always confuses them with my kids. Not because they look alike—in fact, they're not even the same gender—but simply because they don't eat meat, either.)

I am a vegetarian, but it's not because I'm a PETA activist (though I do love little fuzzy critters). And in the beginning, it wasn't even for the resulting benefits to the environment. Nope. It was more likely because for all the wonderful qualities my mother possesses, serving yummy food is not among them. And her meat loaf? Let me put it this way: As soon as my sister and I were old enough to choose our own food, we both became lifelong vegetarians.

Anyway, when my first was born, we lived in Manhattan, and vegetarianism was a really common choice, normal even. We had an amazing pediatrician, a gorgeous Park Avenue doctor who looked like Eva Gabor. She was so glam and superchic she had a Chanel lab coat. I counted on her good advice to point me in the right direction (as did many of the great, glossy parenting magazines). So when my husband and I considered having our baby go sans *carne*, too, of course I wanted Dr. Goldberg's opinion. Her answer? "Why not? She doesn't need meat. No one does."

So this is your opportunity to introduce your child to a healthier lifestyle, for herself and the planet. Even if you and your mate still choose to indulge in an occasional steak or two (it's pretty hard to break the food habits one grows up with), you might want to forgo that option for the little ones. They're starting out with a fresh, clean, and clear palate.

Less Meat Equals Less Angst

To help you embrace your new animal-friendly menu, consider this: According to a recent UN study, eating meat is a greater cause of global warming than car emissions. So switching to non-meat entrées, even occasionally, can dramatically reduce your carbon footprint. Here's another eco-incentive to go meatless. Livestock farming drains huge amounts of precious water from agricultural communities. Each year fourteen trillion gallons go to irrigate fields to produce feed for U.S. livestock animals destined for the dinner table.

I am not on any soapbox, ethically or environmentally. I mean, I may be cutting down on global warming by reducing meat consumption, but only because I've warmed my share with reckless paper usage and happy globe-trotting. I love style magazines and I've probably used enough paper towels to take down ten acres of redwoods. I've flown transatlantically as much as many rock stars (but not, alas, throwing tantrums in first class), and I've never seen a pair of Manolos—animal, vegetable, or mineral—that I didn't think were calling my name. But this is one green thing I've found easy to embrace, for myself, my husband, and my kids: We go veggie all the way.

Cutting down on meat consumption will dramatically reduce your carbon footprint. That's the measure of how much CO_2 your lifestyle puts out on the planet. And CO_2 is what makes for global warming. The U.S. represents only about three percent of the world's population but produces between twenty-three and twenty-nine percent of all carbon emissions. So going meat free in as many meals as you can is more than kind to your four-legged friends—it's kind to us two-legged friends, too!

HELLO, DOLLY

In case you're still not moved to reduce your family's meat consumption, here's one more reason. (Or is it two? Or three? Gosh, they all look the same. . . .)

Ten years ago, the world welcomed the first cloned animal, Dolly the sheep. Now the U.S. has the dubious honor of being the first country to allow meat and milk from cloned cattle into the food supply. The Food and Drug Administration "sees no difference between conventionally raised farm animals and clones. The products of both are equally safe to eat" (*The Guardian*, December 26, 2006).

What kind of protection is in place for the consumer here? Are there any long-term studies of the effects of eating or drinking products from cloned animals?

In a word—NO.

None.

How could there be, when cloning itself is so new? So why are we doing this? What have we got to gain?

There are no apparent benefits to eating cloned meat. And we have no shortage of cows, pigs, and sheep to meet (or meat) current demand, certainly in the developed world. And cloned animals are not an option for many third world countries, who forgo this untested option altogether for the sake of their health and well-being. (As do EU countries, which have either banned the sale of cloned meat altogether or insisted on strict labeling.)

Plus, when greenhouse-gas-emissions specialists tell us giving up a meal of animal meat in favor of veggie counterparts drastically reduces our carbon footprints, why *on earth* are we monkeying around with Mother Nature to make ethically, medically, and economically questionable meat to eat?

Red Flag

Remember, cloning is not a perfect science. Dolly suffered from arthritis and died at a young age for a sheep. Research has since indicated that clones are born with more deformities and other complications.

• • •

Here comes a palate-pleasing road map to animal-friendly eating from the queen of the green, Annie Somerville, executive chef at San Francisco's aptly named Greens Restaurant. And with these savory vegetarian meals, I bet no one will even miss the meat.

Frittata with Caramelized Onions, Goat Cheese, and Sage
MAKES 1 9-INCH FRITTATA; SERVES 8

The flavors of this frittata are wonderfully appealing—the richness of the caramelized onions is just right with the tangy goat cheese and the pungent, earthy sage. A glaze of reduced balsamic vinegar is the final touch—when it's brushed over the warm frittata, its sweet acidity highlights the unusual flavors. You can caramelize the onions a day in advance, but don't be in a hurry. They'll need plenty of time to release their sugars and cook down to a wonderful jamlike consistency.

2 tablespoons light olive oil
3 large onions, about 2 pounds, quartered and thinly sliced
    salt and pepper
3 garlic cloves, finely chopped
8 eggs
1 ounce Parmesan cheese, grated, about ⅓ cup
1 tablespoon chopped fresh sage
3 ounces mild, creamy goat cheese, crumbled
3 tablespoons reduced balsamic vinegar

Preheat the oven to 325 degrees. Heat 1 tablespoon of the olive oil in a large skillet; add the onions, ¼ teaspoon salt, and ⅛ teaspoon pepper. Sauté the onions over medium heat for about 10 minutes to release their juices. Add the garlic; continue to cook over medium heat for about 40 minutes, gently scraping the pan with a wooden spoon to keep the onions from sticking as they caramelize. (Add a little water if needed to loosen the sugars from the pan.) Transfer the onions to a bowl and set aside to cool.

Beat the eggs in a medium-sized bowl. Stir in the onions along with the Parmesan and sage. In a 9-inch sauté pan with an ovenproof handle, heat the remaining tablespoon of oil to just below the smoking point. Swirl the oil around the sides of the pan to coat it. Turn the heat down to low, then immediately pour the frittata mixture into the pan. The eggs will sizzle from the heat. Crumble in the goat cheese and cook over low heat for 5 minutes, until the sides begin to set; transfer to the oven and bake, uncovered, for 20 to 25 minutes, until the frittata is golden and firm.

Loosen the frittata gently with a rubber spatula; the bottom will tend to stick to the pan. Place a plate over the pan, flip it over, and turn the frittata out. Brush the bottom and sides with the vinegar and cut into wedges. Serve warm or at room temperature.

▶ Tip: We always begin cooking our frittatas on the stove, but they can also be cooked entirely in the oven. Combine the vegetables and eggs as directed, but don't add the cheese. Pour the egg-vegetable mixture into an oiled baking dish, then sprinkle or crumble on the cheese. (Adding the cheese at this point keeps it from settling and sticking to the bottom of the baking dish.) Bake for about 25 minutes.

Annie Somerville, Fields of Greens, *New York: Bantam Books, 1993.*

Finn Potato Cakes with Asiago
Makes 12 cakes; serves 4 to 6

Starchy Yellow Finn potatoes are a delightful host for leeks, spring onions, or tender shoots of green garlic and a variety of cheeses. We've chosen Asiago here, but any creamy melting cheese will do; Manchego, Fontina, Gruyère, or chèvre are equally delicious.

The potato mixture holds well in the refrigerator for a day or two, so you can make it ahead of time and cook up the cakes at the last minute.

2 pounds Yellow Finn potatoes
1 tablespoon olive oil

2 medium leeks, white part only, cut in half lengthwise, thinly
   sliced and washed, about 1 cup
salt and pepper
2 teaspoons minced garlic
2 large eggs
2 tablespoons crème fraîche, plus extra for garnish
3 ounces Asiago cheese, grated, about 1/3 cup
1 to 1¼ tablespoons all-purpose flour
oil for the pan

Place the potatoes in a pot of cold water and bring to a boil. Lower the heat and simmer, uncovered, until they're tender but not quite cooked through, about 25 minutes. Drain the potatoes and set aside to cool. Peel the potatoes and grate on the largest hole of a hand grater or in a food processor.

Heat the oil in a medium-sized skillet and add the leeks, ¼ teaspoon salt, and a few pinches of pepper. Cook over medium heat until the leeks begin to soften, about 3 minutes. Add the garlic and cook 1 minute more, adding a little water if needed to keep the leeks from sticking to the pan.

Combine the leeks, potatoes, ¼ teaspoon salt, and a pinch of pepper in a mixing bowl. Beat the eggs and the crème fraîche together and mix into the potatoes along with the cheese and flour.

Form into little cakes about 3 to 4 inches in diameter and ¾-inch thick. Cook in a well-oiled skillet or on a griddle over medium heat, allowing the cakes to crisp and turn golden, about 5 minutes per side.

Annie Somerville, Everyday Greens, *New York: Scribner, 2003.*

Flex It, Please

You don't have to go whole hog (sorry) into the veggie scene. If you or your family feel really attached to meat, you might want to go flexitarian. About forty percent of the U.S. population could be considered flexitarians: people who primarily eat vegetarian but who also eat meat, fish, or poultry occasionally.

ABC, ONE TWO THREE, GMO, GM, GE

"Genetically modified," "genetically engineered," and "genetically modified organisms."

You've probably heard those terms, but who actually has any idea what they really mean? The food giants like Monsanto and Bayer that create, patent, and (believe it or not) in some cases actually *own* these seeds and every one like it (if they have the same DNA) would have us believe genetic modification is nothing more than what we've been doing for centuries—lovingly slicing and sticking together grains just like back in the days of the Pharaohs in order to strengthen crops—so all is swell and well.

But today's genetic engineering is somewhat different from splicing two strong seedlings together and hoping for a better hybrid. It's gonna sound scary, but please don't skip this part; these are things you really do want to know about, since so much of the corn and soy that we eat is genetically modified. About seventy percent of all U.S. corn and ninety percent of all U.S. soy is genetically modified. Eating genetically modified foods has serious implications for our kids, particularly for the staggering number of American children who are food sensitive—one out of three.

Green Guru

Robyn O'Brien
FOUNDER, ALLERGYKIDS

MOM

Meet Robyn, a "plain ol' mom" who morphed into a foodie vigilante (just as the rest of us would do) when one of her kids almost died from food sensitivities. She helped me understand the connection between food production and food allergies. Basically, all our kids run a high risk of becoming "food sensitive" when the food they are eating is so far removed from its natural state. Today genetically modified foods have no labeling in the U.S., and many crops are literally changed, at the DNA level, to include their own pesticide. That means they contain neurotoxins in their very core (no use tryin' to wash that off). Get ready. What she has to say about genetic engineering may change the way you think about every bite.

"A famous French political thinker, Comte de Tocqueville, once said that the public would rather believe a simple lie than a complex truth.

"Genetic engineering has been used for decades to help make crops stronger, and yields higher, but it is only in the last ten years that neurotoxins have been engineered into our food supply. These come in the form of pesticides that are genetically engineered into the cellular data of the organism. A genetic pesticide.

"No one has studied the long-term health implications of children consuming foods containing neurotoxins. But look back over the last ten years and you'll remember that, back then, we didn't have to worry about sending a peanut butter and jelly sandwich into school with our children, we didn't have to medicate our eight-year-olds to get them through the school day, and the movie *Rain Man* was all we knew of autism.

"Today, at least one out of every seventeen children under the age of three has a food allergy, with at least five million American children suffering from this condition. Autism, diabetes, and obesity are often referred to as American epidemics.

"So what changed?

"In 1996, the United States adopted widespread use of genetically modified crops due to growing public concern over the health risks associated with the industrial spraying of insecticidal and pesticidal toxins. In an effort to reduce the spraying of these toxins, scientists began using biotechnology to engineer these pesticides and insecticides into the plants themselves.

"As these ingredients were introduced around the world, government agencies in Australia, Japan, Russia, and forty-five other developed countries required them to be listed on food labels, so that consumers could make informed choices when it came to feeding their families.

"In the United States, however, our regulatory agencies do not require these genetically engineered ingredients to be labeled. So, unlike other developed countries, we have not been informed that almost seventy percent of our corn, ninety percent of our soy, and seventy-five percent of our processed food now contain neurotoxins, novel proteins, and allergens.

"Basically, we have unknowingly and without informed consent engaged our children in one of the largest human trials in history. Today one out of every three children suffers from allergies, asthma, autism, or ADHD. Ten years into this human trial, it appears our children are trying to tell us something."

GENETICALLY MODIFIED: WHAT IT IS AND WHAT IT MIGHT MEAN

The very name is misleading: GM crops are more than modified; they are wholly engineered, created by forcing a strange gene into a complex biological system. They are actually changed in every conceivable way, at the very cellular level. GMOs push us further into a more industrial agricultural model just as we are learning that organic farming and sustainable agriculture provide benefits that conventional agriculture cannot. They also put agribusiness in the driver's seat, as these crop varieties are patented and owned by huge conglomerates.

Finally, and perhaps most important, the effects of genetically modified foods on the biological processes of the human body have not yet been fully understood regarding assimilation, influence on cell states of organs, and aging.

CHILDREN OF THE (POP) CORN

Of all the salty, satisfying no-no's I've banned from the pantry, there is one thing I am not willing to give up—not for me or my kids—and that is popcorn. I sometimes wonder if the Native Americans who introduced the Pilgrims to popcorn ever dreamed how successfully it would become integrated into our lives. For my family, popcorn is actually the staple food it was for the Iroquois. We've spent many a happy evening munching (and arguing over hard-to-comprehend rules) during a game of Scrabble, Clue, or Life. But lately we popcorn lovers have come upon sad and troubling times. Popcorn has turned from the perfect simple snack into a frightening case of Munch at Your Own Risk.

How did this happen?

PFOA (perfluorooctanoic acid) is the chemical used in Teflon pans to make them nonstick. It's also in the coating that lines microwave popcorn bags to keep the corn from sticking to the sides. This is especially important to know when consuming flavored and "buttered" microwave popcorn because PFOAs leach into the flavoring oil. Inhaling the PFOA-laden steam from microwave popcorn, even just twice a day, can put you or your kids at risk of bronchiolitis obliterans, or "popcorn lung," a potentially deadly condition (hardly worth the salty fix).

And it's not just the PFOA that may be at fault. Diacetyl is one of the compounds that gives butter its characteristic taste. Because of this, manufacturers of margarine typically add diacetyl to their products to help mimic butter's appealing flavor. Diacetyl is a common ingredient in butter-flavored microwave popcorn. And diacetyl is also implicated in popcorn lung, to the degree that ConAgra announced that, while its Orville Redenbacher's popcorn is perfectly safe—honest!—they will be removing diacetyl from all their products in the near future.

Add to that the looming question of the safety of genetically modified corn (found in about seventy percent of commercial popcorn) and it loses even more of its appeal. So what's a popcorn lover to do?

Pssst: I've got the good stuff for you, over here. The dealer's name is Steve. (Tell him Lynda sent you. . . .)

Green Guru

Steve Spayd
FARMER
FOUNDER, FARMER STEVE'S POPCORN
FATHER

Sometimes only crunchy-salty will do to satisfy. And usually that means turning a blind eye to health and wellness. But not so with Farmer Steve's Popcorn. And unlike many other yummy treats with folksy names, there really is a Farmer Steve behind the label.

"I farm because I like to grow things. Our farm is certified organic because we want to produce the healthiest food available. With an organic system, our farm uses no chemical fertilizers, no chemical pesticides, and no genetically modified seeds, and our popcorn has no artificial flavoring, partially hydrogenated oils, or trans fats added to it. The final product is as healthy as you can get. I've been farming for eighteen years. I've got four daughters and my second oldest always says she wants to become the 'popcorn heiress,' and I hope she does. Farming organically is a way of life for us. It's a family business for us and we love it."

SAVED BY THE NELL

When is junk food not junk food? When it's yummy, chunky, chocolaty sweet, or salty, savory, crunchy—but really just all-natural. The good stuff—and organic, to boot. Get your hands together for the woman who has won me countless hugs and kisses from my grateful kids as we unpack the grocery bags.

Green Guru

Nell Newman

ORNITHOLOGIST

FOUNDER, ORGANIC DIVISION OF NEWMAN'S OWN

PHILANTHROPIST

Her daddy's rich and her mama's good-lookin' (her dad's pretty good-lookin', too). That combo has been enough to tempt many offspring of Hollywood royalty into a lifetime of poolside leisure and decadent luxury. Not so for Nell Newman, who has added the safe gift of organics to the great food and great work that Newman's Own has been doing.

"My environmental leanings started when I was eight and I learned the peregrine falcon was extinct east of the Mississippi. Now, for a budding ornithologist, that was a staggering moment, understanding the effect mankind could have on the environment, growing food in a way that destroys entire ecosystems and kills the animals and birds that I love. That was the beginning of organics for me. I could see the connection. I knew organic agriculture meant a natural safe haven for all of us.

"The great American bald eagle was devastated by the use of DDT on conventional agriculture. Almost wiped out. DDT causes the eggshells to split, literally running the life right out of them. How sad would it be if we poisoned our national bird to death?

"Predatory birds are like the canary in the coal mine. Birds of prey bioaccumulate contaminants in the environment. They eat small birds and rodents, and small birds and rodents eat the seeds that are these chemical cocktails. That's how the food chain works. And if that's happening to them, what's happening to us?

"The factories and manufacturing plants that make pesticides are all around us. Fifteen years after DDT was banned, we still see the negative effects. Most chemicals eventually degrade in the environment, but some not so well. Many have unforeseen and devastating effects on animals in the wild.

"So as I grew up, I wanted to do something, and I knew organic was a good answer.

"We did our initial research for Newman's Organics in 1993 and 1994; then we launched product in 1994. I was fund-raising for the Predatory Bird Research Group and fund-raising can be really frustrating and ineffective at times. I looked at what Dad was doing and thought, that is interesting—that's a great way to make a difference.

"Our philosophy since then at Newman's Own Organics has been great-tasting products that happen to be organic—

nostalgia foods that remind us of happy memories, like pretzels, which were Dad's favorite food growing up.

"I thought, there's got to be a lot of people out there like Dad who would eat organic if it looked and tasted like what they were used to and enjoyed."

GREEN AT A GLANCE

Evergreen: Educate yourself on the complex (and scary) world of genetically modified foodstuffs and "modify" the foods your family eats to avoid them whenever possible.

Pea green: Plan, make, and eat more meals together. It's loads of fun and much healthier for everyone.

Spring green: Choose organic for the foods your kids eat most frequently. And try to go organic with the foods that have the highest amounts of pesticides when grown conventionally: apples, bell peppers, celery, cherries, imported grapes, nectarines, peaches, pears, potatoes, red raspberries, spinach, and strawberries.

Three 🍃

Green
Home
Improvement

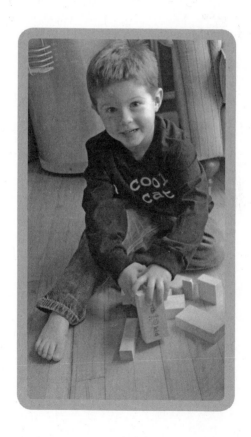

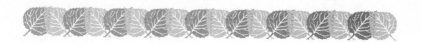

Building the Life You Really Want

My house needs some work—some of it pretty major and some merely cosmetic. Just like practically everyone else in the Western world, I'm a huge fan of *Extreme Makeover: Home Edition* (you can usually find me crying within the first five minutes), and on those rare occasions when my weekend afternoon schedule is cleared of soccer games or kids' birthday parties, I'm happy to settle in for a marathon of TLC's *Trading Spaces* or HGTV's *Curb Appeal*, accompanied by a glass of Pinot Grigio, a big bowl of popcorn, and a pair of cuddly slippers. But, hey, actually DO those things? Me? Oh, I think not. So when the kids grew a little bigger, and we got a little more cash, choosing where and how to begin to fix up our ramshackle house—and stick to our green values—was a complete mystery to us.

Now, when I don't know anything, I let my mind wander.

(I agree with Einstein that imagination is better than . . . well, anything!) So I started dreaming the impossible dream, considering, if I could, how I would redo my house from top to bottom, maybe even build one from scratch. Of course I would need to take into account everything for a true Green Dream House, including

- carbon footprint

- nontoxicity and health

- cost

- natural light

- upkeep

To help my dream take shape in my mind, I looked for, and found, the greatest green-building experts (in the real world, not just in my fantasy), and let them fill in all the blanks.

We haven't built our dream house yet (still happily making do in our romantic old Victorian), but here's what we'll choose when we do.

LEED THE WAY

Wondering who can help you put up that drywall and still stay on your eco-mission? Look for a builder or contractor who is LEED certified. LEED is the nationally accepted benchmark for the design, construction, and operation of high-performance green buildings. The LEED system (Leadership in Energy and Environmental Design Green Building Rating System) was developed by the U.S. Green Building Council in 1998 to encourage the development and implementation of green building practices. LEED certification depends on six categories: sustainable sites, water efficiency, energy and atmosphere, materials and resources, indoor environmental quality, and innovation and design process.

Thinking you might be the only one? According to environmentalist building experts, LEED is one of the fastest-growing sectors of construction today. Check this out from the U.S. Green Building Council:

More than 1,300 commercial buildings are LEED certified.
More than 10,300 commercial buildings are LEED registered (on their way to certification).
More than 500 homes are LEED certified.
Approximately 11,390 homes are LEED registered.

I WOOD, WOOD YOU?

The furniture we spend so much time on, from the sofa in the family room to the beds our kids are sleeping on, usually contains wood, not to mention the floors we're walking on. As basic and natural a choice as wood might seem, from an environmental standpoint, all wood is certainly not created equal.

Green Guru

Bill Ginn

DIRECTOR, GLOBAL FOREST PARTNERSHIP,
THE NATURE CONSERVANCY
AUTHOR

Bill Ginn is the real deal. The uncle of a close friend of mine, Bill has the green cred and a big, big brain. He graciously agreed to get me up to speed on just why we should care (I mean really care, enough to alter our using and buying habits) about the fate of forests, some of which are half a world away, and why recycled-content paper may have a direct impact on our health and well-being. What he gently and patiently explained to me may hold the very key to our survival. Sound overly dramatic? Well, besides being food and shelter to about half the world's species of wildlife, the great tropical rain forests are also the natural world's equivalent of both the drive-through pharmacy and the Clean Air Act.

"One of the most startling things is that twenty to twenty-five percent of all the carbon that's being released into the atmosphere comes from the destruction of forests. A tree is like a giant carbon silo, and when you cut it down, a huge whoosh of carbon is released into the atmosphere. Planting new trees will not bring that back.

"And this is not just happening 'elsewhere'—here in the United States we'll lose forty-four million acres of forest over the next twenty years.

"Ironically, part of the reason the forest has been cleared is to grow soybeans and oil palm for use in alternative fuels. So to solve one problem we've created another.

"The world economy has to acknowledge nature's contribution to human well-being. By rights a developer who offers to buy a forest should be paying not just for the trees but for the costs of damaging the ecosystem.

"Think about the things you buy. Are you buying certified wood? FSC [Forest Stewardship Council] labeling for products is a real thing. Wood is a wonderful material because it is renewable, but not all wood is the same, and not all woods are managed the same way. Only five percent of forests are managed sustainably. We need to demand that all the wood in a lumberyard is certified. Five percent is great, but one hundred percent is where we want to be.

"All of us can use less paper. We can use recycled paper, not virgin. Buying recycled means another tree isn't being taken down.

"We can make protection part of our plan, by supporting the World Wildlife Fund and the Nature Conservancy.

"We can make a difference in our world, but it's not going to happen by accident. People drive the market. It needs to be everyone's job to invest in the future. If we do that, we can make a difference."

THROWING IT ALL AWAY

The throwaway (or flushaway) household staples we just can't live without can be ever so much gentler on the earth if we choose a little more wisely—and they can be exactly the same in terms of price, performance, and convenience, too.

According to the Natural Resources Defense Council, if every household in the U.S. replaced just one roll of virgin-fiber toilet paper with one that was one hundred percent recycled, we could save over four hundred thousand trees.

Check out these other amazing facts from their handy pocket-sized *Shopper's Guide to Home Tissue Products*. If every household in the U.S. replaced one box of virgin-fiber facial tissues with one hundred percent recycled, we'd save 163,000 trees;

one roll of virgin paper towels with one hundred percent recycled, we'd save 544,000 trees;

one package of virgin-fiber napkins with one hundred percent recycled, we'd save 1,000,000 trees.

WHAT YOU CAN DO NOW

1. Buy recycled-content paper products. Some great one hundred percent recycled brands are Marcal, Whole Foods 365, and Seventh Generation.

2. Buy chlorine-free paper products.

3. Support manufacturers that use recycled-content paper products, and boycott those that don't. (See NRDC.org for more easy tips.)

SECOND NATURE
(THE ULTIMATE IN RECYCLING)

If you're in the market for some new furniture, that's great for the economy, and there are terrific craftspeople out there who deserve your support. But the best way to reduce landfill trash and greatly diminish the carbon footprint of manufacturing is to buy used. And there are great deals to be had. (Consider the $15 spent at a local yard sale on a simple side chair that morphed into the $250,000 Early American masterpiece I recently saw on *Antiques Roadshow*. Man! That coulda been me!)

Just be careful. There are some things you really want to steer clear of when used.

Red Flag

Cribs—recalls happen relatively frequently; if you buy one secondhand, you may well have missed a recall notice.

All mattresses—beyond the penta-BDEs (the flame retardants in conventional mattresses that some forward-thinking states are beginning to ban because of their links to cancer), you would be fending off bacteria and possibly even bedbugs—ewwww—OK, I'll say no more!

Pullout sofas—likewise (they have their own mattresses, after all).

Any playthings or furniture for young kids—these are things that are likely to be mouthed, and the older they are, the more likely they are to include lead paint or loose parts.

Pillows—too many yucky things to mention.

Stuffed toys—ditto.

Leaded crystal glassware—lead (duh).

Any remotely suspect ceramics—beware of chips and be suspicious of anything made in China (although a lot is probably OK, a lot is turning up with lead in the glaze).

Green Flag

On the flip side, these are pretty much safe bets:

unpainted furniture
any natural hardwoods

For the best deals check out

- Salvation Army furniture stores

- the local paper for moving/yard sales

- Craigslist.com

SET UP THE SYSTEM TO RECYCLE

With three kids, two dogs, my hubby, and me, we make a lot more trash than I'd like to. One real way to reduce the load that puts on Mother Earth is to add packaging size and materials to the long list of criteria a product gets judged on before I drop it in my shopping cart. Another is to be really vigilant about recycling. Whatever we take into our home either (a) stays there, (b) gets used up, or (c) gets tossed. It's the "gets tossed" category we all want to keep tabs on. Here's some advice from a young cool sage, a total green guy who has some advice about how to get your good green on and keep it on.

Green Guru

Justin Miloro
ASSOCIATE WHOLE BODY COORDINATOR
WHOLE FOODS MARKET

Justin is one of my best friends and a sharp witty soul who knows how to cut through all kinds of holier-than-thou personal greenwashing and the eco-anxiety that comes from always trying to do the right thing. He knows how to choose doable ways to make a difference at the personal and consumer level. Remember, your body and your house are two ways you can start today to green it up.

"What I want to say is that even the littlest thing is going to make an impact. You don't need to dump every single cleaning item you have and replace it this minute—it's not like that. It's a process. Just choose to do your best from this point forward.

"Like now, I don't want to use plastic bags anymore when I shop. So I bought reusable shopping bags. I hang them by the door. I have some in my car. I try to take them with me whenever I go out. I put them in all those places to make it easy for me to maintain this change.

"So that's my philosophy—choose one thing that you want to do and that you can do really well, and watch it make a difference. Do whatever it is that makes you feel good—it should feel good because it *is* good.

"I have two small wastebaskets in my bathroom, one for recycling, one for trash. I realized I was being vigilant with kitchen recycling but tossing shampoo containers when they were empty. Not anymore. It's a simple change, but significant.

"Make one change. Once you get that down, make another."

Green Flag

You probably know that switching to compact fluorescent lightbulbs—those cute squiggly ones that give off the bluish light—is one great way to reduce your carbon footprint. Here's the good news: If every household in the U.S. replaced one incandescent lightbulb with an Energy Star compact fluorescent lightbulb (CFL), it would be the equivalent of removing one million cars from the road (source: www.egov.cityofchicago.org)!

Red Flag
However, CFLs, like all fluorescent lightbulbs, contain a small amount of mercury, and even tiny amounts of mercury are considered hazardous waste. So these bulbs should not go in the regular trash. Go to www.earth911.org and enter your zip code to see the safe disposal options in your neighborhood.

GOT KIDS?
You probably do, or you wouldn't be reading this book. And for all of us, our cuddly kindergartners soon enough morph into temperamental teens (yes, even yours). When that happens, if not before, their room takes on much greater importance. Their ROOM (imagine supernatural glow surrounding the previous word) takes on mythical proportions. And whether it be peppered with purple plush animals or covered with posters of Marilyn Manson, "the room" becomes the center of their universe, and they will probably be spending practically every waking moment there when at home. So when they want to redecorate this extension of their personal aura, the simple addition of a lava lamp probably won't cut it. My friends at Green Depot, *the* environmentalist do-it-yourself home center, have compiled the following tips to help keep your kids' surroundings (if not their language) as clean as possible.

And FYI, when looking for anything home-repair or home-maintenance related, check out www.greendepot.com, the original go-to spot for all things safe and nontoxic for your home.

TOP TEN TIPS FOR A GREEN BEDROOM MAKEOVER

1. **Paint.** Many kids favor dark and bright colors, but these paints are usually very toxic. Paint should be a zero-VOC mixed with zero-VOC colorants. Any caulking should also be low-VOC.

2. **Carpets** should be short nap, tightly woven or tufted, made with nontoxic fibers and glues. Avoid thick, long naps; the fibers are usually toxic and they become breeding grounds for mold, mildew, dander, and dust mites.

3. **Lighting.** Full-spectrum lightbulbs are recommended to reduce eye fatigue and strain from reading, computer work, and TV.

4. **Hardwood floors** should be finished with a low-toxic waterborne urethane to reduce outgassing. An alternative to hardwood is natural linoleum (which has natural-biocide properties) or cork tile, which has natural thermal and acoustic properties.

5. **Beds.** Mattresses and box springs should be made of natural cotton and wool, with no synthetic chemical additives. Encasement sheets that go over the mattress and fit supertight can be used to avoid dust mites, dander, and bedbugs getting into the mattress. (If bedbugs are suspected, use natural chemical solutions to kill them.) The bed frame should be made of metal or sealed woods to prevent outgassing.

6. Furniture. All wood furniture should be completely sealed with either a nontoxic finish or a proper sealant.

7. Air filtration. Consider a portable unit in the room to clean the air of particulates, odors, and gases. You can buy special window screens to eliminate pollens and dust from the outside.

8. Storage. Use hard plastic boxes to store toys, art materials, books, clothes, etc. Cardboard and paper containers are very porous and absorb odors, gases, and mildew spores.

9. Vacuum. Whether you use a canister or upright, make sure it's of the HEPA filter type to ensure that microscopic particulates are trapped in the machine and not redistributed throughout the room.

10. Cleaning products. All cleaning, deodorizing, and laundry products should be of natural formulas. There are so many choices on the market now, this should be a no-brainer switch!

Green Guru

Dennis Johnson
FOUNDER, NATURAL SPACES DOMES

Dome homes look a lot like flying saucers, or big inverted bowls, and they just may be the answer to many of our environmental concerns. In the U.S. sixty percent of carbon emissions (the basis of global warming) come from home energy use. Domes use significantly less of every kind of home energy, from the actual building materials to heating, cooling, and lighting. So opting for one of these modern marvels not only may be key to saving this great green goddess we call home but could put some green back in your pocket, too. And if your neighbors think you landed from another planet, you can truthfully tell 'em, "We come in peace."

"My wife and I live in a dome I built in 1975. It's made from triangles, and it's extremely efficient, materially. A dome uses one-third of the materials that a conventional home of the same square footage does.

"People want domes for different reasons. Some people are chemically sensitive and want to live in a truly green, formaldehyde-free dwelling. Most are attracted to domes because they are so much less expensive to heat, cool, and light.

"Domes make sense everywhere, not just out in the country. We have built domes in the middle of major cities and in dense suburbs. It costs about the same to build a dome as a conventional home. Some parts cost more, but there are savings off the bat, too, and way lower maintenance. For example, if you use high-grade asphalt shingles, they last fifty or sixty years and require zero maintenance. No paint, no trim, no chalk and seal.

"Sometimes people think it's all open space inside, like a giant round loft, but you can have any number of rooms inside the dome. You choose the design that suits your family's needs. We have lots of plans. And it is klutz free, like a big Tinkertoy set. A twenty-five-hundred-square-foot dome shell goes up in two to three days—any builder can do it.

"We have a Dome School twice a year where people come to learn how to put up their own dome. You can have a dome raising, like an old-fashioned barn raising. You may find you've suddenly got a lot of friends. It creates a lot of community and camaraderie, because it's fun and it doesn't take long—you see the results right away.

"I just love what I do. It's fun and engaging to make a positive difference in the place where people spend the most time."

REDUCE, REUSE, REMODEL

OK, if you don't have the inclination—or cash—to build from scratch, but are instead looking to spruce up your existing digs, what's out there? How can you green your home and still fulfill your needs and wants and stay on budget?

The more you look at it, anything new takes resources. A big part of green home design is about revamping and reusing. That means minimal throwaway and also less manufacturing energy.

Let's look at ways to improve your home, and your experience in your home, some of them as free as the air you breathe.

Twenty percent of the U.S. population suffers from allergies, and air quality is an integral part of living the good life you want for your family. Indoor air quality is actually worse in most cases than outdoor air quality—from two to one hundred times worse, according to the EPA. This is partly because Mother Nature has so many safeguards in place outdoors; sunlight and breezes do a whole lot to clean out bad stuff. So the more of each of those you can let inside, the better.

EVERY BREATH YOU TAKE

Follow these tips to dramatically reduce allergens and improve indoor air quality.

- Air out every room in your house every day. Open the windows (even if it's just a little bit on cold days).

- Don't keep room doors closed.

- Pull the blinds up during the day.

- Forgo the use of air fresheners.

- Clean with natural cleaning products, or make your own with vinegar and water.

- Never use pesticides inside or outside the house.

- Opt for natural wood or cement flooring or natural area rugs of wool, jute, or organic cotton.

- Consider an air purifier for where you take the most breaths, like the bedrooms.

- A faithful every-other-day sweeping will work wonders, or use a vacuum with a HEPA filter; it picks up the smallest particles, which are often the worst allergens.

- Do an old-fashioned rug beating. Take area throw rugs outdoors, drape 'em over a laundry line, and whack them with a broom. (The sun will kill millions of dust mites, and a simple breeze will clean and freshen any odors. Plus, the whacking is great for cleaning out your aggressions, too.)

Remember: You don't have to be allergic to adopt these greener habits. You really don't want to be using any conventional cleaning products in your home unless you are sure they are simple, pure, and safe. Because of their chemical cocktail of synthetic fragrances and toxic corrosives, conventional cleaning products are one of the top causes of indoor air pollution.

Here are five lines I love that are very gentle and nontoxic—and that really work!

- Ecover

- Whole Foods 365 Everyday Value Multipurpose Cleaner

- Seventh Generation

- Greening the Cleaning

- BabyGanics

- Green Works

GOOD GREEN CLEAN Is your house a little grungy, yet you're feeling a bit pinched for cash? Don't worry, you've probably already got all you need to do a green clean of your kitchen. Vinegar and water is the perfect replacement for pricey (and sometimes toxic) glass and countertop cleaners. A mix of about one part vinegar to three parts water will usually do the trick. Up the ratio of vinegar if you've got some serious grease to cut, like on a stove top. Avoid using it on marble, though—it'll stain.

Got some gray matter in your tub? A little baking soda on a cloth with a bit of water will buff it right off, no noxious smell and no scratches. Economical, too!

The most important, cheapest (and my least favorite) natural-cleaning secret? A little elbow grease! 🌿

Finally, remember that a huge part of being really clean is to ban any synthetic pesticides from your home and lawn. Adopt preventive measures instead. The Natural Resources Defense Council says, "There are more studies linking the use of pesticides in and around the home, and [pesticide-based] lice treatments, to childhood cancers than anything else."

HOW GREEN IS YOUR VALLEY? Size may not matter, but sometimes placement does. Wanna know how you measure up? Or thinking of a move? Jacob Gordon from Treehugger.com reveals the cleanest and greenest cities in the U.S. by rating them on things like alternative-power usage, ratio of bike riders to cars, climate-protection initiatives, and open space. Here are his picks for the top ten.

Austin	New York
Berkeley	Philadelphia
Boston	Portland (OR)
Chicago	San Francisco
Minneapolis	Seattle

Check out the whole series at www.cityguides.msn.com/citylife/greenarticle.aspx?cp-documentid-4848590. 🌿

GO FOR THE GREEN / SAVE SOME GREEN

Is it possible to have it all? Save some money and save the planet? My husband, who is well-known for his . . . ahem . . . conservation of the kind of paper used to make dollar bills (if ya catch my drift), has practically made a study of some of the most effective ways to save *both* types of green. Here are some of the biggest differences you can make on both fronts.

Go with the (Low) Flow

Twist on a low-flow showerhead and it's likely nobody will even notice. They're designed to reduce water usage while maintaining water pressure. The average family of four can save over two hundred dollars a year.

Put a Sock in It—or a Pair of Jeans

Plug up leaks and drafts. Most homes lose between five and a whopping fifteen percent of their heating or cooling through gaps in doors, loose windows, and such. Plugging these up can be as simple as weather-stripping or caulking. If your attic isn't insulated, you are losing way more. Consider a natural insulation that also frees up landfill space, like UltraTouch, made of recycled blue jeans! It will save you some serious bucks and greatly reduce your carbon footprint.

Be a Johnny Appleseed

Plant a tree on your property (or two—perfect for a snooze in the hammock). Strategically placed shade trees can lower your air-conditioning costs by twenty percent. (Oh, so that's how our grandparents survived the summer. . . .)

Go Solar

Going off the grid—that old-time anarchist movement to get away from paying "the man"—has turned into a reality for many people seeking to shrink their carbon footprint, and shrink their energy bills, too. Sometimes down to zero—yup—Z-E-R-O. The secret? Going solar.

TURN ON THE SAVINGS Converting your home's power source to solar reduces your contribution to global warming—and because electricity is generated primarily from coal, it reduces our dependence on fossil fuels. It also happens to be a shrewd investment. The paybacks come not only in the form of lower utility bills but via cash rebates, tax incentives, and higher real estate values. You may see your full financial return on investment in as little as eight years, depending on which state you live in.

State-sponsored rebate programs can significantly mitigate your initial cost outlay for a solar electric system. The California Energy Commission offers cash rebates of up to $2,800 per kilowatt of system capacity. In Colorado, the rebate is even better: $4,500 per kilowatt—roughly half the approximate $25,000 to $27,000 cost of a 3-kilowatt system. Some solar-electric-system providers will front you the rebate so your initial investment is substantially reduced, with no waiting. Other states—including Alaska, Arizona, Colorado, Connecticut, New York, New Jersey, Pennsylvania, Oregon, and Washington—also have tax incentives and cash rebate programs. (For a full list of incentive programs, visit www.dsireusa .org.)

Plus, with energy prices rising every year, your savings will grow every year, too. Honestly, do you think the cost of fossil fuels is ever going to go down significantly?!

Although it's not necessarily factored into the payback equation, rising real estate values also boost your return on investment. According to the National Appraisers Association, for every dollar of annual energy savings, the value of a home increases twenty dollars. So homeowners who save one thousand dollars a year in electricity costs could see their home's value jump twenty thousand dollars.

Reprinted with permission from www.realgoods.com. Institute for Solar Living.

THREE EASY GREEN OPTIONS NOW

So maybe solar is in your future, but what can you do right now to protect your family and save some bucks on energy and water bills if you're not Ed Begley Jr.? Here are some significant ways to make a difference:

1. Get a power strip for every room. You're more likely to turn off and save electricity if all the computers, cell phones, and Nintendos in the room can be shut off with one click.

2. Invest in a water filter, at least in the kitchen. You will immediately screen out over ninety percent of the chlorine, a chemical linked to cancer. And you may motivate your family to chug more of nature's cure—water. The best? Brita, Aquasana, and Crystal Quest.

3. Caulk it up. If you have a drafty window or two, just do it! Get some caulk and close it up. You're losing money along with that heat. Safecoat Caulking Compound is a nontoxic, water-based, elastic-emulsion-type caulking com-

pound designed to replace oil caulk and putty for windows, cracks, and general maintenance work. It will not dry out or crack and does not release any solvents or obnoxious odors.

HOME IS WHERE THE ART IS

The art of sustainable living, that is. (Unless we're talking *real* art here—maybe you're überlucky and picked up an original Picasso charcoal for a buck at one of those yard sales you've been scanning.) Where we live, and how we live . . . what we enjoy, what we feast our eyes on in our homes . . . can be the framework for what our lives are like outside the home. It can be either a beautiful launching pad or an isolated refuge, but either way, the overall style and aesthetic ambience may be as important to maintaining our health and wellness as all the great green chemical-free things we've been implementing.

Green Guru

Cheryl Terrace
INTERIOR DESIGNER
VITAL DESIGN

Cheryl is an unusual combo of drop-dead gorgeous and endearingly peaceful and good-friend-ish, so people (including me) just genuinely like her. She's widely considered the premier "green" designer in swanky NYC. She's been featured in glossies that range from Condé Nast's *Domino* to *Architectural Digest* (but she's deliberately ethical and tight-lipped about her list of celeb clients). She understands it doesn't take a million bucks to have the home of your green dreams.

"You don't have to go one hundred percent green—that's hard unless you live with a dirt floor. It's simply a matter of finding out what works for your life in a healthy, sustainable, thoughtful way. It's about the impact on your health and the health of the planet. For example, consider the life cycle of a product. I look at how the product was made, where it was manufactured, and what will happen to it in the end.

"Nontoxic equals thoughtful. It's really about honoring home. Treat your home like you treat a person you love.

"Take your shoes off when you enter, so there is a very real separation between the outside world and the inside of your home. Choose beautiful rugs or floors with patina. Offer plants to your home. Instead of buying pesticide-laden roses, get some plants. The oxygen they give off will purify the air, and the energy of a living thing is a gift to your home, and to yourself. If you burn candles, get soy candles, or, even better, beeswax. Burning natural candles is healthy for indoor air quality.

"Decluttering is a huge thing. My advice is, if it's not pretty, don't keep it. Don't accost yourself with stuff. Display a few beautiful things to rest your eyes on. Rest your eyes, rest your mind.

"I want to honor where we live—the planet. Everyone does. If given a choice of nontoxic or toxic, who would ever say, 'Oh, yes, I want the toxic!'

"One day, it won't even be called green; it will just be the way everything is done."

FIVE GREEN THINGS YOU CAN DO EVERY DAY

1. Get beautiful air-cleaning plants like peace lilies or Chinese evergreen.

2. Decorate your home with original art from local artists. You'll be supporting your community and it won't have traveled far, so you'll be reducing your carbon footprint.

3. Take off your shoes at the door.

4. Open the windows, even in winter, for at least a little while.

5. Donate or give away whatever doesn't serve and please you. It may work for someone else and the declutter will calm your mind.

GREEN AT A GLANCE

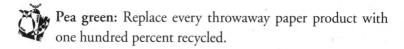 **Evergreen:** Choose a home that reflects your green values (and your low-carbon wishes).

Pea green: Replace every throwaway paper product with one hundred percent recycled.

Spring green: Choose one green thing you can do, and do well, and congratulate yourself—it'll lead to more good green things.

Part II 🌿

Seeds of
Change

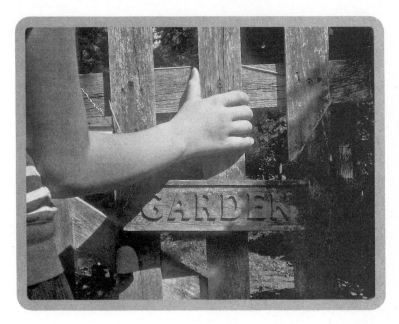

Mighty Oaks from
Little Acorns Grow

What Time Is It? Green Party Time!

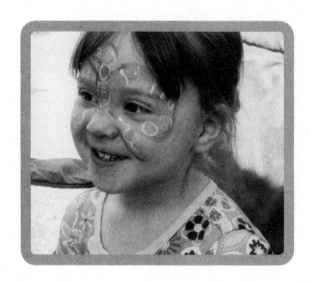

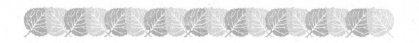

How to Have a Ball Without Goin' to the Mall

You spend a lot of time and effort doing the right thing for your kids and family, so probably your conscious consumerism—the healthful and ethical choices you make in terms of what you buy—has been going pretty well. But now you are about to meet *real* pressure, the heftiest trial and temptation your beautiful, ethical, and growing green way may face (the following to be sung to the tune of "Sympathy for the Devil"): Please allow me to introduce myself, I'm an event of wealth and fame (end cool mental music here).

Yes, it's your kid's birthday party, the biggest exercise in wasteful abandon you're likely to ever have. (OK, except for your wedding, but too late for that now.)

Should you just cave and book that disco bowling party that the apple of your eye has been begging for? Splurge for a Hannah

Montana makeover at the mall for your daughter and her fifteen best friends? Or is it possible for you to do right by your favorite person on their most special day and also do right by the mother of us all, planet Earth?

Parties by their very nature are incredibly wasteful. The wrapping paper alone is an exercise in crazed consumption. If you have one child, you may look forward to this day with high expectations and youthful glee. But if you have more than one, you may be feeling Scroogey, with thoughts like "When will it be over?" and "Do I really have to have all those kids in my house . . . *and* their parents?" But fear not: Parties can still be a celebration (without breaking the bank), and they're the perfect time to venerate what matters to you and what supports your child—our terra verde. As a seasoned veteran of "the birthday bash" (heck, I've thrown thirty-three of them!), I have some advice to dish.

IT'S YOUR PARTY, AND YOU CAN BUY IF YOU WANT TO (BUT YOU DON'T HAVE TO)

First of all, remember, this is actually *your* big day, the day your glorious kid came into being and you became Mama or Papa to her, so you should have it your way . . . the green way. Anyway, you've already done the one birthday that really matters: that first one.

So here's the pep talk. You do not have to succumb to the urge to throw money at the same Build-A-Bear, Chuck E. Cheese, or arcade game room that everyone else is opting for. When you control the environment, it's way easier to keep it green. Plus, from a kid standpoint, there is actually nothing more memorable than a party in your own backyard, kitchen, rec room, or garage. So here's a look at a few of my favorite themes for at-home birthday parties, along with the things you'll need to make them a huge hit.

A Pirate's Life for You

Who doesn't love swashbucklin'? Everyone loves the promise of buried treasure. This is a great party theme for kids of either gender and it's fun for the littlest ones to around age ten.

When we did this one in the backyard, my anti-rain dance worked—the skies opened up just as we waved our good-byes and the garden gate bopped the last little butt and sent the guests on their way.

Here are some ideas, but use your imagination and I bet you'll come up with even more:

In lieu of goody bags, tie up "treasure" in bandannas.
For a cool craft, have the kids make their own eye patches out of black felt and black elastic.
Paint "tattoos" with nontoxic face paint.

WHAT YOU'LL NEED

• A backyard or access to a park

• Pirate's Booty snack (from Robert's American Gourmet) or Natural Cheetos or organic chips

• Stuff for a treasure hunt (colored pencils, wooden tops, a bag of pennies for the ultimate find)

Crafting the Perfect Party

A "make 'n' take" craft can do double duty as a fun party activity and an impressive take-home gift (nixing the need for the standard junk-filled goody bag).

How about a living garden, like an easy-to-grow sunflower in a pot? Provide organic potting mix and let the kids decorate the pots with a good nontoxic craft glue like Aleene's and old buttons or dried peas and beans.

WHAT YOU'LL NEED

• Easy-grow seeds such as morning glories, sunflowers, or a butterfly mix

• Organic potting-soil mix

• Small ceramic pots

• Mixed notions such as buttons, ribbons, coins, nuts and bolts—whatever you have around that you think might look good

• Craft glue or, if an adult will be helping, a craft glue gun (watch it, though—the glue gets HOT!)

Green Olympics

If you want to get them running around, this is the theme for you. Unless you have a hip loft or a palatial mansion, though, you'll need to do it outside. A park or town green will work if you don't have a backyard. Have a beanbag toss where guests make their own beanbags out of socks and dry rice. (Put the rice in individual cups the kids can pour into socks; then have them just tie off or knot the ends.) Set up laundry baskets or old coffee cans for the targets. Three-legged races and sack races (you can use old pillowcases) are always a huge laugh, as are spoon-and-egg races. Here's another old favorite, the shoe race: Have everyone take off their shoes and put them in a big pile. A member of each team runs to the pile, finds and puts on his or her shoes, and runs back to tag the next person.

WHAT YOU'LL NEED

• Clean socks (finally a use for all those single socks!)

• A big bag of dry rice or peas, lentils, etc.

• Laundry baskets or coffee cans (the older the kids, the smaller the targets can be)

• Pillowcases or burlap sacks for the sack race

• Tablespoons and eggs (hard-boil them first if you want to avoid a mess, though for some people that's the whole point!)

LET THE GAMES BEGIN

Remember, kids love games, regardless of where you hold the party or what your theme is. You don't have to reinvent the wheel. Tried-and-true classics like Pin the Tail on the Donkey, Hot Potato, and Duck Duck Goose let kids be their exuberant selves, and they can easily be tweaked to fit your theme.

Another advantage is that they aren't too wildly competitive. Take it from one who's learned the hard way: It's usually happier for everyone if the party games are focused on the doing rather than the winning. Every child should "win" and the prizes should be basically equal.

Musical chairs can be a haven of happy, healthy hysteria for tweens and teens if you choose of-the-moment music and let them keep their own tempo. For parties where space is tight, charades is full of fun.

There are lots of Web sites out there with fun, and free, games and crafts. Check out www.ivillage.com or www.planetgreen .com.

Whatever you choose, please remember how lucky you are,

and that there's no right or wrong. You have your kid; you are on the planet; this is a day to really celebrate. P.S. If your wonderful kid is less than stellar at her happy event, who cares? Chances are, she came into this world on her first birthday crying, too.

Green Guru

Tiffany Washko
WRITER, NATUREMOMS.COM
MOM

Lest you feel alone, I have found another mom who has mulled over the conundrum of the eco–b-day party with great ideas and wisdom. Meet Green Guru Tiffany Washko.

"I don't think anything has a natural mom cringing more than the thought of a conventional birthday party. It generates enormous amounts of garbage, the kids are hyped up on sugary birthday cake, and they get lots of toys that frankly they just don't need.

"Fortunately, having a green party is easier than you might think. Let's start with invitations. There are quite a few choices for eco-friendly birthday invitations nowadays. You can use invitations made from recycled paper, of course, or seeded invitations, which are embedded with a mixture of annual and perennial wildflower seeds. There is also the tree-free paper option. Tree-free paper is exactly what it sounds like, paper that is made without *any* cuttings from trees, directly or indirectly. Instead the paper is made from more sustainable materials. You can always make your own invitations out of scrap paper you have at home.

"Now, on to presents. Well, I don't know about you, but my kids already have too many toys, on top of which many gifts will be made of plastic that's full of toxins and chemicals that can have harmful effects on children. Plus, plastic breaks quite easily, and then because it's nonrecyclable, the toys end up in landfills. So maybe you could request on your recycled invitations that guests bring your child a used book or a gently used toy from their own home. Many parents would appreciate this.

"Consider suggesting on the invitations that all gifts be wrapped in newspaper or fabric. The newspaper can be recycled and the fabric can be reused for a variety of other things."

MORE TIPS FOR A GREEN PARTY

• Use reusable dishes, utensils, and napkins. All these can just be washed instead of being tossed.

• If you MUST use disposables, then go for the Preserve disposables, available at Amazon. They are made from recycled yogurt cups. You can also buy compostable utensils.

• If you do have any plastic, aluminum, or glass waste at the party, set out labeled recycling bins for the guests and encourage the kids to use them.

• Instead of a plastic tablecloth, use cloth. If you have your heart set on a themed tablecloth, see if you can find a similarly themed sheet.

• If you're giving out goody bags, ditch the plastic and go with fabric there, too.

THE POSH NOSH

What's a birthday party without sweets? Of *course* we want to let them gorge a little on their special day. I really believe it is not the sugar that has most kids bouncing off the walls but the synthetic flavors and colors. So for party classics with a healthy spin, here are some sweet sensations.

The best chocolate cake ever (I swear!) comes from Cherrybrook Kitchen and is totally vegan. I know, it sounds unbelievable, but try it, and you'll be a convert. Plus you can whip it up as easily as a conventional mix. Available at Whole Foods or www.cherrybrookkitchen.com.

Another great choice, and this one's organic to boot, is Goodbaker chocolate cake and cupcake mix—rich, organic chocolate-cake mix that's vegan but tastes as good as a junky mix.

One good tip: Remember, the younger the child, the easier it is to dictate the exact foodstuffs you'll be doling out. Use your lordly power! Jelly on little corners of bread or yogurt sprinkled with raisins can be surprisingly well received by the kids, and a huge relief for parents when picking up little ones after the shindig is over.

If you do choose to go classic, cupcakes are OK, but you may want to have kids make the icing themselves, out of confectioners' sugar and water. They can top it off with berries. Give each guest a small bowl of berries to drizzle over the cupcake (works well on sponge cake or pound cake, too). The colors are pleasing and the naturally sweet flavor of the fruit is super satisfying, with none of the scary, makes-'em-hyper fake colors.

A WISH COME TRUE I shudder to think of all those colorful bits (and bites) of wax from melted birthday candles my kids ingested before I learned of the toxins involved (regular candles are made from petroleum). Beeswax candles are the ultimate in green party cake toppers. Go for Big Dipper Wax Works birthday candles, about five dollars a pack.

UP, UP, AND AWAY

One of the most eye-pleasing decorations (which often does double duty as a goody at the end of the party) is, unfortunately, one of the biggest eco-taboos: balloons. Perhaps you've heard the sad stories of manatees and dolphins found asphyxiated because they mistook a balloon for their fave treat, a jellyfish. When I heard that, I immediately switched to the more expensive but luxe-looking and long-lasting silver Mylar balloons. But, lo, those are no better for Mother Earth. The average Mylar balloon will take five hundred years to biodegrade. So better to opt for more earthbound decor, like Chinese lanterns.

IF YOUR KID IS ALREADY A BUDDING ALBERT SCHWEITZER Some kids seem to be born deep thinkers. In our house we don't watch the news in front of the kids, so they don't have a handle on how really bad it can be for some other folks. However, my middle one always had some amazingly admirable Angelina Jolie leanings anyway. She has manned many a fund-raising table with me, exhibiting the zeal other kids reserve for the opportunity to collect the latest Webkinz. So when it comes to her b-day, we opt for some philanthropic endeavors. Here are some of the best.

Instead of traditional gifts, you might ask family and friends to contribute to a pool of donations and give a goat, chickens, or even an ox to an Appalachian family in need. Check out www .gardenharvest.org.

You can donate directly to kids who are missing the greatest joy, a family, by choosing the button *Donate now* on Worldwide Orphans Foundation's Web site at www.wwo.org.

Or, if you want to split the joy (and the loot), you might consider a new resource called ECHOage. According to the site: "An ECHOage birthday party is a unique opportunity for you and your child to do something extraordinary—to improve the world—together. Here's how: Guests are invited to an ECHOage birthday party online. Instead of bringing a wrapped and packaged present, guests simply RSVP and give a secure online gift of money. Payments are pooled for the purchase of ONE special gift and to support ONE meaningful cause."

Your kid surfs the site and chooses whom to donate to from among their prescreened charities. I admit this seems like a really cool idea to me; note, however, that they pocket fifteen percent off the top. With a little research, you may be able to set up the same kind of thing yourself, without losing such a substantial chunk.

'TIS THE SEASON

Having kids means the calendar is filled with other days to celebrate, too. Formerly overlooked holidays take on a previously unforeseen significance (and, of course, another reason to buy stuff). Valentines must be doled out to classmates, and a driven—sometimes almost sacred—gusto surrounds the Halloween costume. Later in the year little folks can be quite vocal about what Santa is meant to bestow upon them, since they have been very, very nice (you knew that at some point you'd pay for that surprise A+ in English)!

So how can we make everyone's dreams come true and also ensure a Very Green Holiday?

Let's take a quick run through the red-letter days on the calendar and how to keep them green.

Be My Homemade Valentine

A batch of cookies wrapped in parchment and tied with jute can be a welcome and wholesome treat for the teacher or for the entire class. If you're not up for Suzy Homemaking, you can buy organic candy or invest a little time in the class by bringing in a story and reading to the kids. After a heartfelt discussion about the nature of consumerism, and the real nature of love, my astute little one came up with the following one year: In lieu of traditional valentines, she made a fill-in-the-blanks poem for each of the kids and I keyed it into my laptop:

The nature of love is _____
The love of nature is _____

And we left another line for the poet's name and date.

This project required very little paper because we printed the poem nine times on each sheet and then cut out each one to glue onto pretty scrap paper. We decorated the poems from our stash of "pretty things": buttons, bits of ribbon, yarn, cards, and gently used wrapping paper. If you have a stash like this, pull it out (and if you don't, consider making one in an old shoe box or the like—you'll be amazed at the creations that can be brought to life from repurposed "junk"). If not, construction paper will do.

Every child got a unique valentine, thanks to our "pretty things" box, and I'm virtually certain they didn't get tossed at the end of the day, either, but instead were kept as a beautiful reminder of our connection to one another and to the earth.

A Very (Very) Scary Halloween

Now let's look at big fat holiday number two. In the U.S. Halloween comes in a close second from a financial-expenditure standpoint after Christmas and Hanukkah. (I somehow knew it wasn't Mother's Day.) And Halloween means a whole lotta junk. Junk food, junk decorations, and sometimes even downright dangerously junky Halloween costumes.

Most of the stuff used to decorate your house (and your kids) for Halloween is made of polyvinyl chloride, or PVC. PVC outgasses phthalates, an endocrine-disrupting chemical that acts as a faux estrogen, feminizing boys and womanizing girls far earlier than normal. This is probably not the image change our kids were looking for as they donned their scary new duds. And it's in just about every conceivable add-on of the Halloween experience, from the much-mouthed (and therefore ingested) fangs to the Freddie Krueger mask on your kid's precious noggin.

I have craftsy kids, so they usually embrace the idea of home-made costumes. These typically consist of clothing we already own and a little bit of artfully applied makeup, so they're super inexpensive and easy on the environment.

There are some great online resources that can show you how to make your own costumes at home, and many from stuff you already have. Check out www.budget101.com/hw1.htm. This one is incredibly comprehensive—my eight-year-old chimes in, "It's AWESOME!" And I can pretty much guarantee your kids will find a bunch of choices they love, too. The accompanying pix look amazing and many of the costumes are pretty easy (for those of you who are craft challenged). They compile the choices from a bunch of different sites and also have real characters (Scooby-Doo, X-Men, etc.), if your kids have their hearts set on a known image.

My youngest used the same black leggings and dress for two years in a row, first as a black cat, and the next year as a little witch; the only change was a headband with ears (for the cat) and a store-bought hat for the witch. These were stunning, though, because of the black eye pencil that gave her whiskers and an inverted-triangle nose one year, a blacked-out tooth and heavily lined eyes to make her a riveting witch the next.

Keep in mind, you really want to use the best-quality makeup, because most of the "nontoxic" greasepaint sold (especially around Halloween) contains high amounts of lead. No, it's not supposed to, but with the millions of products pushing through our borders fighting for shelf space around this time of year, it's unlikely the offenders will get found out.

Choose really clean and trusted brands from health-food stores like Whole Foods Market or holistic pharmacies like Pharmaca, or get Burt's Bees, which is available at just about every corner drugstore. CVS has some natural stuff, too—please, *please* don't buy anything from dollar stores. . . . They are highly unregulated and there must be some reason they are trying to dump it so fast and cheap. If you really go green for Halloween, you'll be avoiding more than lead; chances are, you can sidestep potential carcinogens like parabens and allergens like synthetic fragrances, too.

MY FAVORITE BRANDS OF MAKEUP

- Dr. Hauschka

- Lavera

- Zia Natural Skincare

- Aubrey

PLAY FAIR (TRADE, THAT IS) If you're in a hurry, Global Exchange can give you a guilt-free hookup for the holiday. It's the only fair trade, ethically produced Halloween kit I have ever seen. For fifteen dollars you get the following:

- A bag of Equal Exchange fair trade chocolate candy to hand out to trick-or-treaters (forty-two individual pieces)

- A large stack of festive Halloween postcards for you to hand out (these are great for teacher greetings)

- Traditional *papel picado* Mexican party streamers

- A trick-or-treat bag made from recycled Kraft paper decorated with a friendly Fair Trade ghost

They've got kits for Valentine's Day and Easter, too (www .globalexchangestore.org). 🍃

With all the opulence and shenanigans rolled out before our gremlins, the simple orange Unicef box is a gift for kids less fortunate, and a great gift to our kids, too. I love that they tell you right on the box specifically what the money can accomplish. Not only does it encourage math skills as the kids count the loot they collected, but it can inspire great generosity. I know that after checking out how far five dollars goes, my frugal eight-year-old was moved to raid her own piggy bank. Even the little ones understand it really is better to give than receive!

THIS LITTLE LIGHT OF MINE For trick-or-treating, I suit my kids up with shake 'n' light flashlights, powered not by batteries but by—you guessed it—shaking. Hey, they've gotta work off those candy calories somehow. Great to have around the house for any power outages, too. You can get them at www.realgoods.com. 🍃

Have a Very Fair Trade Christmas

Right after Thanksgiving, when the stores open at four a.m. and some of us are sharpening our elbows to get down and dirty for the best sales, somewhere deep inside, we may also be contemplating a better way. Now, I am not talking about giving up buying—I love my stuff, to give it and to get it. But could it be that we can get the great goods and make the world better at the same time?

Fair trade is the way to go. Fair trade means a living wage or better for the craftspeople, artisans, and farmers in developing countries who grow or make the goods we choose.

And what better way to spread goodwill than to celebrate the season with something that helps others. Besides, the craftsmanship of fair trade goods is especially beautiful because the people who make them aren't under the gun of oppressive management or slave-labor conditions.

Here are some great sources:

- www.worldofgood.com

- Global Exchange (freestanding stores and online)

- Ten Thousand Villages (freestanding stores and online)

Pig Out

What to buy for the person who REALLY has everything? How about an ox or a pig? Heifer International will take your financial gift and purchase a portion of an animal, or even an entire animal, depending on the size of your gift, and give it to a family in need in the name of whomever you choose. And lest you think this is just for hippie-dippies, it's a favorite of gorgeous superstar Susan Sarandon. (OK, so maybe she is a hippie, but a very glamorous one!)

Oh! Christmas Tree

If you want a really green Christmas, think not just about what's under the tree but about the tree itself.

In case you think you're going green by opting for a real tree over the perfect-looking plastic one from Kmart, you're half-right. Unfortunately, along with the fresh smell of pine, you are likely bringing in a chemical cocktail in the form of potent herbicides and pesticides (many of which are banned from foodstuffs). So as little ones are decorating the tree, they may be spreading more than good cheer. I know it's sad to think about, but unless it's a certified-organic tree, this is what's happening in your living room, thanks to your poison-laden Christmas tree.

At http://www.ecobusinesslinks.com/organic_christmas_trees you can look up organic Christmas tree farms. There aren't too many of them (the closest one to where I live is three hundred miles away), but maybe you'll get lucky!

Another option is a live tree in a pot from a green nursery. Even if they're not certified organic, trees that are being sold alive as opposed to cut are sprayed much less with toxic chemicals, so you won't be putting your family at the same risk by bringing one inside. After the holidays you can replant it outside. Keep in mind that, depending on where you live, the ground may be a little less than yielding for the shovel, so you may want to

1. dig early, before the frost, then cover back in with a topping of bagged organic soil;

2. choose a small tree, four feet or under, so the roots don't need to go so deep. Plus it's fun for the kids to watch it grow year after year (just like them!).

If you do opt for a conventional Christmas tree, please consider bathing little ones after the decorating.

Seeing the Light

In the past few years you might have noticed that there are increasing numbers of Christmas-tree lights marked LED. Well, last year I did what I thought was a very ignoble thing: Instead of spending the better part of a weekend afternoon swearing under my breath as I tried to untangle the old tree lights, I tossed 'em and bought all new LEDs from Home Depot. I felt horribly guilty until I learned that I was actually doing the planet (and my bank account) a favor.

"LED" stands for "light-emitting diode," a ditty that translates into lots of light using very little electricity—about ninety percent less electricity than regular bulbs. Not only are the LED bulbs inexpensive, but the portion of your electricity bill allotted to holiday lights will be about ninety percent cheaper. They also give off very little heat, so the risk of fire is greatly reduced.

You're still going to have to wind them up neatly when the holiday is over, though; they last about twenty years. And that's a job that should be yours alone, not the kids'. All the Christmas-tree lights I can find contain lead in the wiring; it's used as a softener in the plastic coating to keep it pliable. Don't let your kids help you place the lights, even when they are unplugged, and be vigilant about washing up thoroughly after you do it.

IT'S UP TO YOU, NEW YORK, NEW YORK Leave it to New York City's innovative mayor, Mike Bloomberg, to find a way to turn the most famous Christmas tree in the world a deeper shade of green. The giant Rockefeller Center tree now features thirty thousand LED lights powered by solar panels. The energy saved by using LEDs as opposed to conventional lighting is enough to power a two-thousand-square-foot home for a family of four for a month. And that's not all. When the season is over, the tree is milled into lumber for Habitat for Humanity.

Candle, Candle, Burning Bright

Of all the candles lit in millions of homes during the holiday season, Hanukkah candles hold a very special place in the hearts and homes of observers, a glowing symbol of the miracle being celebrated. But because of the amount of time Hanukkah candles burn, you'll want to be especially careful about just what they are made of and opt for natural candles like soy or, even better, beeswax. Conventional wax candles are made from petroleum and can actually heavily pollute the air. Even worse, some candles have metal wicks (to keep the wick from flopping over and going out in the wax). University studies show burning as few as two metal-wick candles for three hours can pose "a significant threat to human health," especially for the very young and very old.

To make your celebration a healthy Festival of Lights, the Jewish Museum has a huge selection of ivory, honey, or multicolored beeswax Hanukkah candles at www.jewishmuseum .org.

GREEN AT A GLANCE

Evergreen: Forgo conventional gifts for birthdays or the holidays and sponsor an animal for World Wildlife Fund or give an animal through Heifer International or Garden Harvest.

Pea green: Outsource as little as possible for your kids' shindig. You'll have a lot more control over the ensuing waste; plus it'll be much more memorable for them.

Spring green: If you've gotta go fast and furious, opt for one hundred percent recycled-content disposable paper products and wash-or-toss disposable utensils made of bamboo or corn, which biodegrade safely.

Five 🍃

School
Rules

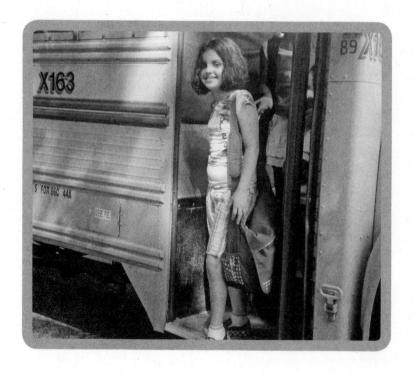

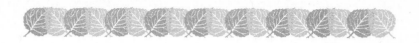

How to Green Up Your Kids' School

Jump rope, tag, first crushes, best friends . . . school is such a huge part of our kids' lives—and so looked forward to by us parents when September rolls around! I vividly remember scouting preschools in Manhattan for my first, Layla. Which one would be good enough, safe enough, challenging enough—but not too demanding!—for my wonderful kid and her growing brain? I needed a preschool that would inspire greatness in my potential Rhodes scholar, my future Nobel laureate, not for me and the reflected glory, but for her and her phenomenal potential. I'd been warned to start the process early (it's very competitive there—think Prada sample sale) and I didn't have a ton of dough, to boot, so I began informally looking when she was only a year old, and then in deep earnest when she turned two, even though I knew she wouldn't actually start until she was three. I bet those think-ahead frantics sound like weird first-time-mom stuff, but it worked; I found a great preschool (and it was even—almost—within my budget)!

Anyway, if your tyke is little, I bet you are on the hunt, too. And don't worry, one day you'll look back at these stressful days with the warm and fuzzy feelings usually reserved for your grandmother's chocolate-chip cookies or a Thomas Kinkade painting. But for now, you may want to add a few more things to your growing checklist of must-haves in a preschool or day care situation. These come from developmental psychologist turned green-school pioneer Dr. Lisa Ecklund-Flores, director of the Church Street School for Music and Art in Manhattan.

Ask your potential school if they can or will do any of these:

1. Use environmentally friendly cleaning and janitorial products

2. Serve organic snacks and juices at snack time

3. Teach children through the art curriculum to reuse "trash" creatively, and encourage them to bring in items from home, such as milk jugs, egg cartons, cardboard, and paper

4. Participate in outreach programs that encourage responsible environmental behaviors, such as "Bash the Trash," which teaches children to make working musical instruments from discarded household items

5. Develop administrative practices that encourage electronic communication rather than paper notices, thereby reducing the amount of paper consumed

6. Use paper products with the highest recycled content possible

7. Recycle paper, plastic, and other applicable materials

8. Work with a green building-supply company to ensure that the materials and finishes that will be used for any construction or expansion will be environmentally responsible, from natural linoleum and no-VOC paints to mold-resistant drywall and a high-efficiency HVAC system

Dr. Ecklund-Flores has put all these into practice at Church Street School over the past year during their "Go Green" initiative. She says, "It doesn't have to be all-or-nothing, and it doesn't have to be all at once, but it's so worth doing. Any school really should have a green plan."

YOU'RE A BIG KID NOW

Every birthday is an incredibly joyous occasion, a milestone for your child. But the fifth birthday often brings with it more than the usual celebration. Five makes for the magic of kindergarten, and for most parents that means a huge shift. If you're the primary caregiver and a stay-at-home parent, your day just opened right up. If you have full-time child care, you're probably going to rethink that arrangement and the resulting money you pay out. Lots of things are different when your child begins spending so many hours of his week at school.

For most kids in America, kindergarten means entering the public school system. Here's some stuff you may want to be aware of as your child enters this public domain, and what you can do to keep your kid in the pink (and green).

THE WHEELS ON THE BUS

I always tried to encourage my kids to ride the bus. I wanted them to feel independent, and I figured it was probably good for them socially, too. Plus, it's a huge time-saver for me, walking them to the bus stop instead of carting them back and forth to school, and from an environmental standpoint, driving them when there is already a bus scheduled to pick them up ranks somewhere between thoughtless and downright irresponsible.

However, as we look further, this choice becomes as muddy as the sky above a coal-burning power plant.

According to the Web site of the nonprofit watchdog Environmental Defense Fund:

> Yale University studied the air quality inside buses by attaching monitors to children's backpacks and recording the pollution levels during their trips to school. Levels spiked when buses arrived to pick them up, remained elevated on board, spiked again as they exited the bus, and returned to low levels upon entering the school.
>
> While children may only spend a few hours per day on school buses, the high levels of exposure encountered on board school buses can add considerably to their daily and annual exposures to air pollutants such as [diesel particulate matter] and PM2.5.

Red Flag

Kids are getting MORE exposure ON the bus than around it—five to six times more than outside. This may constitute a significant hazard to your child's breathing, most certainly if the child already has asthma. According to the California Air Resources Board, "school bus trips can increase children's daily exposure to black carbon up to thirty-four percent compared to regular passenger cars. Particle levels inside a school bus can be five to ten times the levels outside the bus."

A University of California study found, "The total mass of bus pollution inhaled by bus riders likely exceeds the total bus pollution inhaled by the [entire] remaining public, despite bus riders being a relatively small group." (For more information visit www.environmentaldefense.org.)

Green Flag

There is a simple and relatively inexpensive solution: With a simple filter retrofit onto the exhausts of old-style diesel school buses, we could immediately reduce the dangerous emissions by seventy-eight percent. The cost? About seven hundred dollars per bus, a small investment considering the impact it can have on our kids' health.

What to do? Any decent-sized public school system has a transportation department. You may want to check in with them and hear if they have any plans to retrofit the buses in your district. If not, bring it up at the next PTA meeting. I was really surprised to see how few people knew about this huge danger to our kids. Now we are on the way to the filters.

SAY IT, DON'T SPRAY IT

According to a July 2007 story in the online journal Science-Daily, "More than 80 percent of schools in America use toxic pesticides as a preventive measure, whether it's needed or not."

The story goes on to say,

> Mark Lame, an entomologist and professor at Indiana University's School of Public and Environmental Affairs,

believes this is an entirely unnecessary practice that carries more risks than benefits to students and faculty.

"The most widely used pesticides are, in fact, nerve poisons. They cause uncontrolled nerve firing, and disrupt the delicate hormone systems. The link between pesticide exposure and health problems in children is already well established. Research has connected these endocrine-disrupting pesticides to health problems such as ADHD, autism, and infertility—all of which are on the rise."

So what can you do to limit your child's exposure to these toxins?

Call your district's administration and (politely) ask what the school policy is on pest management. Do not settle for a well-meaning but general "We almost never spray" or "It's all state approved." Remember: It is your right to know, and besides, this is potentially the biggest favor you can do for your entire community. Childhood cancer is at epidemic levels in the U.S. and still rising. Cancer is the number two killer of American kids, and besides home, which you are already making safe and healthy for your child, school is where she will spend the most hours of her day.

Here's a step-by-step plan that you might want to use. It'll keep you from losing your cool (this is not the time to be one hot mama) and help you protect your kid.

1. Find out exactly what the school is using. Get the actual names of the products and ask for specific procedures like "wait time" between the application and kids' being allowed to reenter the building, play on the fields, etc.

2. Check out your findings with the master of safe bug bait, Beyond Pesticides at www.beyondpesticides.org, or do your own research online.

3. If the news is bad, don't freak out! Sing (quietly), "I've got the power," and download stats from the CDC (Centers for Disease Control) to back up your concerns.

4. Go back to www.beyondpesticides.org and print out their easy-to-understand work sheets about integrated pest management procedures (IPM) to give to the powers-that-be.

5. Make an appointment with the school's superintendent and present your (and your kid's) case.

6. If you get stonewalled, KEEP YOUR COOL and arrange to make a speech at the next PTA meeting. Sadly, just about everyone's lives have been touched by cancer, so it's likely you will have some serious support by the end of the evening.

Final thoughts, based on my own insipid rambling at such events:

• Keep it super short.

• Don't get personal about any miffs you have felt from school personnel.

• Keep it upbeat—"power to the happy civilized people" and all that. Very few peeps really want to be revolutionaries.

• Stick to the facts and don't shriek or cry, even though the stakes are so high for all the kids.

Good luck! And if you make great progress, please shoot me an e-mail at mail@greenbabies.com. *¡Viva la revolución!*

AMERICA'S NEXT TOP ROLE MODEL

Mr. Chips, Annie Sullivan, Gabe Kotter, Ana Rios. The most influential person in your kid's world is, surprisingly, not Miley Cyrus, Derek Jeter, or any one of the smiling *High School Musical* clan, but his teacher. With the low pay, long hours, and high stress, you can bet most teachers really like kids and have their best interests at heart. You don't always win the lottery, but when you do (as in the case of Ms. Rios, above, my Nadia's third-grade teacher), you know they've got your kids' back, and your kids' ear, so as they are igniting our children's desire for knowledge, they also have a golden opportunity to give some good green guidance.

Green Guru

Tessa Hill
FOUNDER, KIDS FOR SAVING EARTH
MOM

Tessa is a beautiful, articulate, warm, and funny woman who really gets how kids think, and what they're interested in. A former teacher and mom of two, Tessa embodies the good green life. Her son, Clint, founded the nonprofit Kids for Saving Earth, and when he died at the age of eleven from nongenetic cancer, Tessa carried on his dream and vision and made it accessible to kids everywhere. Kids for Saving Earth (KSE) provides free environmental-education curricula by mail and online. Conservation, endangered species, rain forests, toxic-waste sites, health issues, and many more ecological concerns are covered on the Web site. My savvy (and highly critical) kids LOVE the material, so it really is speaking their language.

"Teachers can do so much to foster what works (or not). Everything in the classroom is multiplied, so if you really want to make a difference, take it to your child's classroom. Children remember—we all do—what we hear and experience in school. So we developed an action guide to make the environment part of the curriculum.

"The *Kids for Saving Earth Action Guide* has age-appropriate activities from first grade through high school. There are also lots of ideas online on our site and elsewhere.

"Kids love events, like an eco-carnival or a used-book sale. One of our most popular fund-raisers is the soda club—make your own pop! That way you control what goes in.

"Make suggestions or just let them choose their own call to action, to decide what's important to them, and make a commitment.

"I was a teacher for seven years, so I know what kids can do. Often they learn and educate their parents! As we say at KSE, Earth Day should be every day!"

Check out an enormous amount of kid-pleasing classroom activities at www.kidsforsavingearth.org.

SCHOOL OF THOUGHT

As green is sweeping the country and becoming a national priority, it's happening especially quickly in publicly funded places like state and federal buildings and parks, and, in particular, schools. Though it may not seem like a lot can be done about older school buildings in terms of energy and resource conservation, in reality, schools are a great place to start cutting back our carbon emissions, for two reasons.

First, there is tremendous waste in most public buildings, including schools, from paper usage to lights left on unnecessarily, to computers and other equipment that aren't powered down. Second, wanting our kids to have better lives than ours (cornerstone of parenting) means giving them the knowledge—and the power to act—that we might not have had growing up.

Besides, you're never too young to start pondering the big questions, such as "When do I have enough?" and "What does 'away' really mean when I throw something away?" Give kids a chance. With their nimble minds and healthy bodies, they can probably solve a lot of the problems that we didn't even know we had until now. So let's get our thinking caps on and head off to school.

Green Guru

Meghan Fitzgerald
ASSISTANT PRINCIPAL, WASHINGTON IRVING SCHOOL,
WESTCHESTER COUNTY, NEW YORK

At this middle school in Tarrytown, New York, Meghan is chairing the newly formed Green Committee for the district. Tarrytown is a beautiful spot, but it's not exactly Berkeley or

Woodstock in terms of enviro leanings. So what Meghan is accomplishing is not only beneficial for her area but probably going to make sense where you live, too.

"I worked in Internet tech in San Francisco and got involved in environmental issues out there, but I was drawn to teaching, so I left Yahoo to teach math and science. After five years of teaching in California, I moved back east. Schools in different places have different issues when it comes to the environment, but one thing that works everywhere is resource management: managing what the school uses, better. That's an accessible point to start for both the community and the school.

"We started with paper, because it is so expensive, both in cost to the taxpayers and cost to the environment. Across the whole district we're asking, what kind of paper do we use, and what percentage of recycled content is it? Even if recycled paper costs more, if we reduce our usage through better resource management, can we maintain the same cost? And at the same time we're opening up the conversation to kids about how to recycle every day.

"Here are three steps that are easy to implement in any school:

1. Have a recycling bin in each classroom to separate papers from other trash.

2. Teach kids the three Rs—Remind, Reuse, and Recycle—and have them participate in getting the message out. Have

them come up with 'ads' in creative writing and posters in art class.

3. Have the kids take turns being their classroom's Energy Guards, turning off the lights when children leave the classroom, putting computers to sleep, reminding their classmates to use the recycling bins.

"Part of our paper-reduction plan was to make all school announcements and bulletins, which we used to send home in the kids' backpacks, available electronically instead. So parents can opt out of the paper system (just like you do with junk mail) but get the info via e-mail or online at our Web site. We figured out it saves 1,200 to 1,800 sheets of paper every week! So it has a pretty significant impact.

"My favorite green move that we're doing here at Washington Irving is also the most fun: During morning announcements over the loudspeaker, we now include a 'green tip of the day.' Yesterday's tip came from a fifth grader: Place Post-its on every light switch that say 'When not in use, stop the juice!'"

A final note: If you want to offer a meaningful incentive to your school district (whose budget may already be feeling a little overburdened), consider this. According to a September 20, 2007, *Time* magazine story entitled "Little Green Schoolhouse," "Sultana High School in San Bernardino, CA, used basic conservation techniques, like shutting off lights and equipment when not in use, to cut its energy bills by $100,000—half of which Sultana was allowed to keep for its own use."

IT'S ALL IN YOUR HEAD

The pet you swore you'd never have is the one that has a gazillion babies, six legs each, and lives on your kid's head. . . . Welcome to the downside of "It takes a village!"

When my Mina started fourth grade, she developed a weird pattern of twitching and scratching. She's a middle child, and frankly, I figured it was a means to get attention (one of many psychological insights I gleaned from years of watching Jan on *The Brady Bunch*). I took her to the pediatrician to rule out anything physical, which he did, and then he asked if she was under any stress. Dang! She had always seemed so confident and nonchalant, but that had to be it. I made an appointment with a very expensive shrink for my newly troubled kid.

Meanwhile, my girls were looking rather shaggy, so I took them for a haircut at the swanky salon where my friend Kathy works. I dropped them off and went to park my car. When I returned, my young-uns were loitering outside the salon. "Hmm, that's strange," I thought, approaching. . . .

"They're filled with nits," said my gorgeous friend the hairdresser.

"Huh?" said I.

"They have head lice."

"What????"

"Oh yeah," she answered. "They're both infested, and you probably are, too. Come here, let me take a look. . . ."

It all fades to black from there.

May this never happen to you. But if it does, please, please, do not go the conventional route of pesticide-based lice shampoo!

There are serious risks associated with the use of conventional lice shampoos, especially for children. In many states, the jury is not even out on this, and conventional lice shampoos are not available over the counter anymore. If they are still available where you live, *don't buy them and don't use them.* I know, many of us busy parents assume that if it's on the shelf of the local store, it must be OK. If not, wouldn't it be taken off the shelves? Aren't there laws to protect us from dangerous products? Unfortunately, mounting scientific and medical evidence proves otherwise. Remember that only a few years ago DEET was widely available and parents were slathering it all over their kids to keep the bugs "Off." It took a long time for the regulations to catch up to the science.

The EPA admits, "There is no safe level of pesticides," just those deemed to be a lower risk. But when the risk is childhood cancer, I don't think "lower" is really low enough.

The CDC states that there may be a connection between the pesticides used in chemical lice shampoos and nongenetic childhood leukemia, and there are many recent studies supporting this connection. Look at the conclusion of "Non-Hodgkin's Lymphoma in Children Linked to Pesticide Exposure," published in *Cancer* (Dec. 1, 2007): "In utero and early childhood exposure to pesticides is associated with a significantly increased risk for developing non-Hodgkin's lymphoma (NHL)."

And it's not only cancer. Most pesticides are neurotoxins and endocrine disrupters that work by attacking an insect's ability to reproduce. Some studies show that in the long term they may be doing the same to us. Further, a recent study shows a possible link between autism and certain pesticides.

Some of these pesticides are the exact same ones found in the best-selling lice shampoo on the market—the only lice shampoo I found on the shelves of my town's chain drugstore. Lice shampoos are poisons that you don't even need a prescription for. We should not be putting them on our kids' heads!

And why should we when there are alternatives? Hair Clean 1-2-3 (available at most natural-food stores and holistic pharmacies and endorsed by the public school system of California) is effective and does not contain these pesticides. You can get it at www.drugstore.com or www.evitamins.com.

If you choose to go ahead with the conventional treatment, despite the risks, you know what? It might not even work. Unfortunately, it is becoming more and more evident that lice have developed a resistance to the products intended to kill them. Repeated use only complicates the situation and puts your child at further risk of exposure to these toxic chemical products.

Here's a better plan for what to do if the unwanted guests take up residence, based on recommendations from the American Head Lice Information Center. Note: *The most important thing is to get out all the nits.* One nit left behind can create a whole new problem. When removing lice, always work under a good light.

Step 1. Start with the natural head-lice-removal system endorsed by the California public school system, Hair Clean 1-2-3, available at Whole Foods. Spray it in, massage it into your child's scalp (it smells OK, like licorice), and leave in for fifteen minutes.

Step 2. Wrap your child in a towel and sit her on the edge of the tub. Dry shampoo her hair with ordinary shampoo. Pop her into the bath or shower to rinse. Squeeze excess water out of the hair and wrap her up again in a towel and sit her on the edge of the tub.

Step 3. Pour a LOT of any thick white hair conditioner on your child's hair and section some off with a clip.

Step 4. With a lice comb (included in the Hair Clean 1-2-3 kit or purchased separately from a drugstore), comb through the hair in about half-inch sections, working from the scalp to the ends. Flick the conditioner off the comb into a bowl or into the sink. Continue through the whole scalp, occasionally running water through the comb. Yes, this is time-consuming, but you don't want to rush it. It should take a half hour to forty-five minutes to do it right. (You may want to run warm water in the bath for your child's feet if she gets cold.)

If your child does have head lice, you will find the actual lice (which are either dead from the treatment or very slow from the conditioner) or the tiny nits.

How to recognize the little buggers?

Lice are very small and usually pale to medium brown; they look like a sesame seed (with legs! aahhhhh!). Nits will be gray and even tinier, like a piece of dandruff but hard to pull off the hair shaft.

To see if you're getting any out, occasionally comb through the blobs of conditioner in the sink—according to a recent Harvard University study, most people will never have more than seven live lice at any one time.

Step 5. When you are done combing, have your child rinse the excess conditioner out in the shower and towel dry her hair. (Segregate the towels for a superhot wash and dry.)

Step 6. Blow-dry your child's hair on high until it is fully dry. (Recent Harvard studies suggest hot air may kill unhatched eggs.)

Step 7. Put your child's hair up or in a tight ponytail to prevent anyone else in the family from getting infected.

Step 8. Before bed, massage olive oil into your child's hair and scalp, then cover with a shower cap to minimize the mess (you may also want to put a towel over her pillow). Boil the comb before using it again, whether on the same child or another family member.

For two more days, repeat steps 2 through 8. If on day three you see NO nits or lice in the conditioner comb-out, have your child checked by the school nurse to see if she can return to school.

Finally, *whether or not you think your child is lice and nit free, repeat all steps 1 through 8 after ten days*—this is the incubation period for the eggs.

Oh, and in case you think I'm dirty trailer trash, consider the huge outbreaks of both bedbugs and head lice throughout Westchester County, New York, home of Martha Stewart, Hillary and Bill Clinton, and a whole lot of other movers and shakers. Having lice is not now and never has been an issue of hygiene or socioeconomic class. And these days, the pesticide-resistant kind is so strong—darn that Darwin—that they may soon be coming to a head near you. So judge not, and don't worry—if my phobic self can live through it, so can you. We just have to keep our heads . . . and keep our kids' heads away from these toxins.

GOING TO CELL IN A HANDBASKET

I've got a piece of information that might make that big fat NO at the cell phone store a whole lot easier! Here goes: Your cell phone might cause brain cancer. (And no, I'm not receiving this message via crop circles. . . .) In the middle of 2008, two major warnings were issued against kids and cell phone use, first from the Canadian government, followed by the Pittsburgh Cancer Center. Prominent cancer specialist Dr. Herberman of the University of Pittsburgh Cancer told the Associated Press, "Really at the heart of my concern is that we shouldn't wait for a definitive study to come out, but err on the side of being safe rather than sorry later."

In a memo to staff and faculty, Dr. Herberman suggested:

• Children should use cell phones only for emergencies because their brains are still developing.

• Adults should keep the phone away from the head and use the speakerphone or a wireless headset.

• Cell phones should not be used in public places such as a bus because it exposes others to the phone's electromagnetic fields.

First secondhand smoke—now secondhand talk?!

Cancer authority Dr. David Servan-Schreiber, a brain researcher, brain cancer survivor, and author of the international bestseller *Anticancer: A New Way of Life*, had this to say when I asked him to sum up his thoughts on kids and cell phones: "Children under twelve should not be allowed to use a cell phone unless it's an emergency. We already know from studies of adults that an hour a day for more than ten years doubles their risk of brain cancer on the side of the head they use the phone. And we know that cell phone radiation penetrates the brains of children radically more than the brains of adults."

As if that's not bad enough, other studies link dramatically reduced semen count and . . . uh . . . activity to cell phone use. According to a joint study conducted by Reproductive Research

Center, Glickman Urological Institute and Department of Obstetrics-Gynecology, and the Cleveland Clinic Foundation:

> "Use of cell phones decreases the semen quality in men by decreasing the sperm count, motility, viability, and normal morphology. The decrease in sperm parameters was dependent on the duration of daily exposure to cell phones and independent of the initial semen quality." (PubMed.gov and the Associated Press)

France and India have cautioned against children's use of cell phones, but in the U.S. the FDA is staunchly denying the risk from cell phone radiation. It's up to us parents (and bill payers) to curtail their use for our kids—or cut it out all together. Good luck. This is going to be one tough battle!

TURF WARS

OK, now I'm going to get myself in hot water with a bunch of folks in my town—and perhaps with my husband, who is the regional commissioner for AYSO, the American Youth Soccer Organization. But I'm going to risk it and share this one with you anyway. Like many families, we spend a lot of happy hours watching our kids play soccer. I admit I'm a rather lame soccer mom; my kids never have matching socks and their teammates dread when it's my turn to bring the snack. I usually choose organic strawberries and water instead of M&M'S-laden granola bars and blue Gatorade. Plus I've been heard to cheer wildly no matter which team scores a goal—hey, you have to applaud effort.

But none of that is to say I don't care. I care a lot. And I'm very worried that when it comes to our town's growing desire for better fields, most parents of sports-playing kids are pushing for artificial turf.

Most people think artificial turf is better for the kids, and cheaper and easier to maintain for the town. Unfortunately, promoters' claims that artificial turf is a cost-efficient, environment- and user-friendly product that can replace natural grass on sports fields are often unsubstantiated and usually highly questionable. Here are just a few of the problems.

• Artificial turf frequently outgasses volatile organic compounds (VOCs). This is of special concern for children, who are more sensitive to emissions, and for the rapidly growing number of Americans with asthma.

• Ground tire rubber is used in some artificial fields as an impact-softening base. The toxic content of tires (including heavy metals) makes it against the law to toss them in the regular garbage or dump them in landfills or waterways. So why would want we this (in large quantities) where children and professional athletes come into direct contact with it?

• After a recent game my daughter played on another town's artificial field, there was a trail of thousands of little black specks all over our house about half the size of a peppercorn. By the way, we have a strict policy of shoes off in the foyer, so these specks weren't even from my little Beckham's shoes; they had come in on her socks, clothes, or hair. That's a lot of exposure, both for her on the field and for anyone here at home.

• Temperatures on artificial turf have been documented to be eighty degrees hotter than on natural-grass fields under identical conditions. The faux "grass" that looks green to us looks black (due to the ground black tire refuse) when viewed from above, and that's just the way the sun sees it, too. In actual studies, when the natural-grass surface temperature was 93.5 degrees (Fahrenheit), the measured artificial-field temperature was 180 degrees (Fahrenheit)!

• Herbicides, fungicides, and algicides are not labeled by the Environmental Protection Agency for application on artificial surfaces because of fears of runoff and contamination, but these same chemicals are being used anyway on some and maybe most synthetic fields. After all, they are outside and do fall prey to wildlife and pests.

Purveyors (i.e., profiteers) of artificial turf would have us believe that their stuff is much safer for our kids to play on than grass, that it's a veritable jumpy castle in terms of cushioning falls and protection from the resulting injuries. But this is actually not well documented. Many of the "success stories" involve comparing artificial turf with really badly maintained and lumpy natural fields, ones with gopher holes and such.

Plus artificial turf has opened up some new hurts: "Turf toe," a painful condition similar to a stubbed toe times a gazillion (that's scientific doctor talk), is at an all-time high. Though turf toe can occur on any playing field, it happens most frequently on—you guessed it—artificial turf. And the abrasions and contact burns that occur in sports played on artificial turf are much greater than those that occur on natural grass. This is a big issue in sports in which the uniform does not fully cover the limbs. (Like, uh, soccer.)

So, in the question of natural grass or plastic, decide what you want to do, whom you want to play with, and what you want your kids exposed to. But consider, what real good can come from a plastic and toxic outgassing coat that covers large areas of outdoor spaces? Spaces your kids are spending a lot of time breathing and playing on? What about all the toxic trash being carried around your house and town by innocent cleats and sneaker treads? And finally, who actually pays for those seductive studies that say artificial turf causes fewer injuries and costs less "in the long run"? As great as a low-maintenance, perfect-looking field sounds, the beneficiaries might not be your town or your kids. Maybe it's the makers and sellers of this "modern miracle."

When we think about going green, for us, for our kids, for our planet, it really doesn't make sense to take some of our most used wide-open spaces, and cover them with a layer of toxic refuse and plastic.

GREEN AT A GLANCE

Evergreen: Join a green committee in your school district, or start your own! Work to keep your fields growing, green, and natural.

Pea green: Support your child's teacher and take advantage of the good green works that are there to help, such as Kids For Saving Earth.

Spring green: Look for a school that is working to reduce toxic exposure for your kids, whether by serving organic snacks or maintaining pesticide-free fields.

Six 🍃

What's for Lunch?

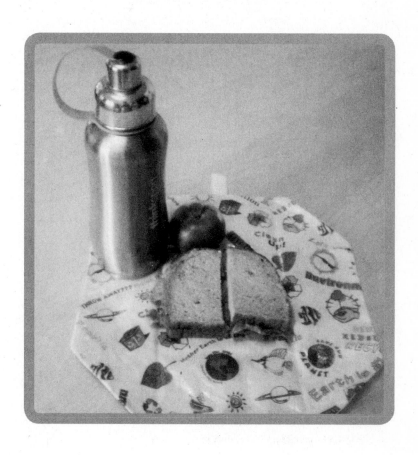

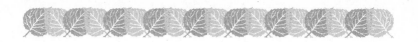

Opening Pandora's Lunch Box

Every morning during the week I get up at five forty-five. Not for a noble run to keep my blood pressure down (and my tush up), nor to dash to the morning train to commute to work. Not even for a quick downward dog and sun salutation, to help ensure my little corner of peace on earth.

Nope, I am up before the rooster crows to make my kids lunch, so they can avoid the school cafeteria food.

Mentally planning, buying, and then actually assembling (by the light of the moon) the fifteen school lunches I pack each week is fraught with the anxiety formerly reserved for a 1950s home-maker faced with hosting a dinner party for her husband's boss. Everything . . . must . . . be . . . just . . . right.

Don't get me wrong. I am not some striving Stepford mom. Rather, I believe—I know—that if my kids avoid certain foods, and consume certain others, they'll be more focused, do better in school, and be healthier.

SCHOOL DAZE

I'd like to be diplomatic, but I'm just gonna cut to the chase here.

Our kids are not doing well in school.

I think they are under the influence of something chemical.

They are ingesting dangerous mind-altering substances, things that were never intended to enter the human body.

And they're lining up in the cafeteria to get them.

Unfortunately I am not joking. . . . School food is making our kids stupid.

And if it's not rendering them actually stupid, it is most certainly getting in the way of them reaching their highest potential.

And we are literally paying for this predicament.

We taxpaying parents feel justified in demanding improved textbooks and school facilities, but sometimes we just don't get what a huge impact the school lunch menu has on our kids' chances for academic success.

The school food system put in place, nobly, by President Harry Truman was meant to protect kids who didn't have enough to eat at home. And the menu hasn't changed much. Unfortunately, a lot of other things have.

Back in the dawn of school-lunch time, foods were calorie laden because many kids were malnourished; they simply did not consume enough calories to get them through the day. Not so today! In the U.S., obesity is more of a problem than malnourishment, thanks to the calorie-laden, low-nutritive corn syrup solids in so many foods made for kids.

In the old days, there weren't any dangerous chemical preservatives in school lunches because food didn't need a long shelf life; it was prepared right in the school kitchen, the same day it was eaten. Not so today. Today's school lunch might be made months, even years, before kids eat it, then sealed up, and locked away, with much of its flavor and nutritive value stripped from it. And the ingredients may come from places as far-flung as China and a host of other countries, making transparency and traceability somewhere between unlikely and impossible.

In the old days, milk was free of rBGH (bovine growth hormone), meats weren't irradiated, genetic modification was not accomplished with a gene-splicing gun, chicken was not liberally sprinkled with MSG, and French fries were not fried in oil laced with BHT. Not so today. Today, school lunch food is a combination of frozen, reconstituted "foodstuffs" that contain such a battery of chemicals that most of us would be hard-pressed to pronounce, let alone recognize, the ingredient listings.

Welcome to the next generation, and twenty-eight million schoolchildren in the U.S. are eating these lunches every day.

FOOD FOR THOUGHT

In the 1970s, Elizabeth Cagan was the New York City public schools' chief administrator. She reversed the trend of the new chemically laden lunches and required the meals served in the city's eight hundred schools to have

- no artificial coloring or flavoring

- no nonbeneficial additives

- no carbonated soda

- only pure fruit juice

- whole wheat buns for hamburgers and hot dogs.

Dr. Stephen Schoenthaler documented the dramatic rise in test scores as a result of the changes in the food in New York City schools. Despite the fact that there was no effort to change what the students ate outside school, their test scores rose from the thirty-ninth percentile on the California Achievement Test (CAT) to above the fifty-fifth percentile (source: www.school-lunch .org).

Overall, across the board there was a fifteen to eighteen percent rise in standardized test scores—and the only change was what the schools served for lunch.

Eventually Ms. Cagan moved on, and her protective and progressive ideas went with her. Too soon, kids in New York's public schools were exposed to the same chemical cocktail kids all over America were. And we are living with those results today: markedly lower test scores and a rising rate of obesity in younger and younger children.

The Centers for Disease Control (CDC) calls childhood obesity "an epidemic." It's estimated that one in three kids born in the United States after the year 2000 will become diabetic in his or her lifetime. For the first time in recent history, the CDC says, our kids will not live as long as we do, and diet is the number one reason why.

MIND YOUR Ps AND Ps There's a great rule that can help protect our kids, especially as the scientific data on toxins are emerging so quickly. It's called the precautionary principle. Here, the nonprofit Science and Environmental Health Network explains succinctly just what it is:

When an activity raises threats of harm to human health or the environment, precautionary measures should be taken even if some cause-and-effect relationships are not fully established scientifically. In this context the proponent of an activity, rather than the public, should bear the burden of proof. The process of applying the precautionary principle must be open, informed and democratic and must include potentially affected parties. It must also involve an examination of the full range of alternatives, including no action. (Wingspread Statement on the Precautionary Principle, Jan. 1998) The precautionary principle, virtually unknown here six years ago, is now a U.S. phenomenon. In December 2001 the *New York Times Magazine* listed the principle as one of the most influential ideas of the year, describing the intellectual, ethical, and policy framework SEHN had developed around the principle. In June 2003, the Board of Supervisors of the City and County of San Francisco became the first government body in the United States to make the precautionary principle the basis for all its environmental policy.

That only makes sense. Let's implement the very reasonable and doable "Precautionary Principle," otherwise known as "better safe than sorry." 🍃

AM I BLUE?

Childhood depression and anxiety are on the rise. And numerous studies now suggest that those blue feelings may be coming from blue food coloring. And red, and yellow . . . The chemicals in fake food have side effects. In a very real way, we are implicating our kids in a massive chemical-burden test, a living, breathing human guinea pig experiment.

Commonly used food additives may affect behavior. You wouldn't give your kid a beer for breakfast and then wonder why he scored badly on a test, but in many ways that is just what we are doing, serving kids chemical time bombs in the form of "nutritious" lunches. We know that thirty percent of the U.S. population is MSG sensitive, with side effects that range from dizziness to lack of focus to fainting, yet there is no ban on MSG in school food; in fact, it is one of the most ubiquitous additives. We know American kids suffer exponentially from ADD, ADHD, and other attention-related disorders, conditions that have been shown to be triggered and heightened by exposure to commonly used synthetic food colorings and preservatives. Yet these additives have not been banned from school food. On the contrary, you are more likely to find higher concentrations of these additives in the low-cost, low-value, long-life foodstuffs served to our children in the school lunchroom than in any of a number of fast-food restaurants.

THE LAND OF MILK AND MONEY In New York State, the law requires an eight-ounce serving of milk with every tax-subsidized school lunch. That means a carton of milk on every tray with every lunch served out of public school cafeterias, wanted or not. Aside from the horrific waste this represents, much of this milk comes from cows treated with rBGH (bovine growth hormone), which is administered so cows produce more milk in less time. That's great for the dairies and for the maker of rBGH, Monsanto. Not necessarily great for the cows, and definitely not for us. There have been no good studies of the long-term effects of rBGH in humans, and there is certainly no nutritive benefit. In fact, in some studies it is linked to obesity and cancer. Bovine growth hormone is completely banned in Germany, and clear labeling is required in the UK. Why are American schoolchildren being given it regularly, without labeling—and why are schools pushing it on our kids?

With all the budget cuts and all the supplies needed for our kids, removing the mandatory milk carton might be a great way to begin to balance the budget.

The overall chemical burden on American children is unprecedented, without comparison in the rest of the world. Environment-related illnesses in children—including asthma, cancer, ADD/ADHD, allergies, and diabetes—are at an all-time high. And the eventual onset of infertility and Parkinson's is not the legacy we wish to leave our children. They deserve better than this, and our society does, too. We owe it to this generation of kids to find a pathway out of this chemical wasteland, and one of the easiest and fastest ways is to just say no to Frankenfood.

Here's the top-ten list for better school food (reprinted with permission from BetterSchoolFood.org).

1. Eliminate all products containing partially hydrogenated oils. Trans fats increase harmful LDL cholesterol and decrease good cholesterol, which can contribute to heart disease.

2. Eliminate high-fructose corn syrup. High-fructose corn syrup (HFCS) has a high glycemic index and converts to fat more than any other sugar. It increases the risk of type 2 diabetes, obesity, coronary heart disease, strokes, and cancer. Americans consumed on average 62.6 pounds of HFCS in 2001, according to the USDA. Many of the products on the market containing HFCS are geared towards children.

3. Pay attention to portion size. Researchers have found that portion size matters as much as taste when it comes to overeating. A recent study showed that large packages and containers prompted people to eat more than the actual recommended serving size regardless of taste. These oversized packages can be especially confusing to children, who may not look at nutrition labels regarding varying portion sizes—especially worrisome because children and teenagers are getting a greater percentage of their calorie intake from snacks.

4. Serve more fresh fruit and vegetables. Many U.S. schoolchildren are consuming more calories daily than needed, as well as choosing foods and snacks that are low in nutrients. In order to achieve normal growth and development of children and to reduce the risk of various chronic diseases, nutrient recommendations must be linked to keeping calories under control. With nearly fifty percent of the calories of children being consumed outside the home, it is imperative that schools offer nutrient-dense foods such as fresh fruit and vegetables in order to obtain the USDA daily recommendations.

5. Support local farms/set up farm-to-school programs. Farm-to-school programs, through which locally grown foods are served and promoted, are beneficial for a number of reasons. Fruits and vegetables sourced locally are fresher, so they taste better, resulting in kids eating more of them. The purchase of locally grown foods supports the local economy and strengthens the local food system. Farm-to-school programs allow students to learn about, as well as appreciate, the sources of the foods they eat and to understand the importance of local agriculture. Farm-to-school programs benefit the environment by cutting down on the amount of fossil fuels used to transport food from the farm to the consumer.

6. Offer vegetarian options daily. As the quality of mass-produced animal protein sources comes under scrutiny based on the amount of residual antibiotics, hormones, steroids and saturated-fat content, vegetarian meals are wholesome options to be incorporated into school lunch on a rotating basis. Institutional foods, as purchased by many schools, may not always provide the most wholesome sources of animal protein. Vegetarian meals, not only wholesome and nutritious, also tend to be more economical, assisting the food budget.

7. Serve more whole grains and beans. The body needs carbohydrates mainly for energy. The best sources of carbohydrates are whole grains because the body cannot digest them as quickly as highly processed carbohydrates. This keeps blood sugar and insulin levels from rising, then falling, too quickly. Better control of blood sugar and insulin can keep hunger at bay and may prevent the development of type 2 diabetes. Eating whole grains may also make kids feel more satisfied for a longer period of time.

8. Discontinue use of poor-quality oils. Partially hydrogenated oils used for frying and food preparation, which are usually industrially processed oils such as soy, corn, cottonseed and canola, are derived from genetically modified food sources and extrapolated into oil using high heat and chemical processes, thus denaturing the oil and making it difficult to be utilized properly by the body. This phenomenon is linked to many diseases.

9. Give adequate time for students to eat lunch. Students need adequate time to eat to meet their nutritional needs, which is essential for optimal student health and performance. Students who aren't rushed can relax, make healthier food choices, and enjoy their food more. Food served but not eaten does not contribute to nutritional health. Allowing enough time for students to eat can also prevent transient hunger that hinders attention and learning.

10. Decrease refined-carbohydrate foods and snacks. Highly refined carbohydrates are rapidly absorbed into the body, much like simple sugars, resulting in a spike in glucose levels. This causes individuals to still feel hungry or to become hungrier sooner, only to consume even more food. This repetitive pattern is believed to contribute to the obesity epidemic. It also increases the risk for type 2 diabetes and heart disease.

Green Guru

Amy Kalafa
MOM
FILMMAKER

Meet a mom who took her fight to school—and won. Producer Amy Kalafa lives in a swanky district in Connecticut and was shocked to learn that her daughter had tempting access to Rice Krispies Treats, Pepperidge Farm Goldfish, and assorted chips every day as part of her middle school lunchtime experience. Amy got mad and decided to look further at what was going on in school lunchrooms, and how it could be improved. She documented her exciting, funny, and sometimes frustrating journey in the film *Two Angry Moms*.

"Back in 1986 I founded the first organic poultry farm on the East Coast. We did it because my husband is French, and frankly, we couldn't find any food that was the same quality he was used to eating. It was great. We supplied the finest restaurants in this part of the world. But we were considered weird, even deviant!

"My kids usually went to school with a bag lunch, so I didn't give school lunches much thought. Finally I woke up. I suddenly realized this is important for other people to know. I am going to make a movie about better food in schools.

"Healthy food is food grown in healthy soil without toxic chemicals and served in a state close to its original form. This 'enhanced' school food has a longer and longer shelf life, which means it is made to not break down easily in the environment—but what does that mean inside our bodies? The whole issue of obesity is only one result, the one we can see most easily. But others are lack of focus and irritability, to name just two more.

"We need to understand, it's not about reading the menu—it's about knowing every ingredient. My goal is for parents to get together. We can change things! It's fixable, we have the tools, and our kids are worth it.

"I kept meeting parents who had taken the first exciting steps to better health for their kids—they had formed groups to study school food. But when I went to search for schools that had actually made changes, I really had a tough time. They always eventually ran up against the same arguments from the food-service producers:

• It costs too much.

• The kids won't like it.

• We can only use USDA government surplus items (i.e., leftovers).

"Those are the standard answers from school providers. But don't give up; it can take time to get your voice heard. Remember, as Yale professor Kelly Brownell says, 'There is a lot of nutrition education going on in our schools, but it's being done by the food industry. Billions are being spent.' So it may take a while for your 'new' view to break through.

"I eventually met Dr. Susan Rubin, the founder of Better School Food, and the two of us became the two original Angry Moms. I filmed her for a year in her school district in Katonah, New York, and the huge and healthy change that district made is an inspiration. They now have access to a salad bar, fresh fruits and veggies, and we successfully banned most of the high-fat, low-nutrition snack foods."

SWITCH FROM FAKE TO FOOD!

Instead of:	Choose this:
Kool-Aid	**Juice, water, sugar**
Jell-O	**Unflavored gelatin and fruit juice**
Cheetos	**Natural Cheetos**
Sunny Delight	**Orange juice**
Fat-free Miracle Whip	**Original Miracle Whip**
M&M'S	**SunDrops**
Hershey's bar	**Ghirardelli bar**
Froot Loops	**Kellogg's Crispix**
Hawaiian Punch	**Minute Maid Fruit Punch**

(Source: www.school-lunch.org.)

ALL WRAPPED UP

So maybe you feel empowered and have decided to try to take on the school powers that be. Or maybe you realize you don't have the time or the stomach for the big food fight and (like me) opt to sidestep this hot potato (sorry—couldn't resist) by sending your kids to school every day with a lunch from home. All right, there's nothing wrong with that. So, what shall we send, and how shall we send it?

You're probably way cleverer in the kitchen than I am, but even I can come up with a week's worth of quick homemade lunches.

Monday

Peanut Better Sandwich

- Organic peanut butter with a choice of a sprinkle of cinnamon or a thin layer of organic honey on whole wheat

- Organic apple

- Organic cheddar slices and crackers

- Iced herbal tea

Tuesday

Olive You Pasta Salad

- Fusilli or bow tie pasta in simple sauce you made the night before of olive oil, fresh roasted garlic crushed in salt and parsley flakes, salt and pepper to taste

- Organic soup in a thermos

- Organic raisins

- Organic lemonade

Wednesday

Avocado, Cheese, and Thank You Sandwich

- Fresh sliced avocado on whole wheat bread with mayonnaise and a slice of Organic Valley Swiss cheese

- Farmer Steve's Popcorn

- Whole Foods 365 Everyday Value chocolate-chip cookies

- Filtered tap water in a reusable bottle

Thursday

Chili sans Carne

- Veggie burger fast fried in olive oil with a sprinkle of garlic salt and chili powder on a toasted whole wheat English muffin with a dash of ketchup or marinara sauce. (This is yummy even when cold thanks to the "heat" of the chili spice.) Top with a bit of fresh spinach, which keeps the sauce from making the muffin soggy.

- Organic banana

- Natural granola bar

- Iced herbal tea

Friday

The Besto Pesto

- Cheese tortellini or cheese and spinach tortellini in store-bought or homemade pesto

- Organic precut and washed baby carrot sticks

- Nature's Promise raspberry vanilla cookies

- Organic apple juice

Homemade Pesto Sauce
(3 TO 4 SERVINGS)

1. Roughly chop 2 cups fresh basil in the food processor. Remove.

2. Combine in food processor ⅓ cup olive oil and 13 walnuts (add a few pine nuts if you want to be authentic) and pulse until chunky.

3. Add ⅓ cup grated Parmesan (you could use some Romano, but it has a lot of "bite" for some kids) and pulse.

4. Mix with the basil.

▶ Voilà! You're a chef extraordinaire!!

TRAVELING LIGHT (GREEN)
So, what's the best way to send that super lunch you just made?

Here's the simple math: My 3 kids times 180 school days equals

- 540 single-use plastic water bottles

- 1,080 fold-over plastic sandwich bags for snacks and sandwiches

• 1,080 paper towels wrapping the above to keep food from coming into direct contact with the phthalate-leaching plastic bag.

Eventually I decided to rethink the packaging, and here's what I came up with, some meaningful and money-saving solutions.

SIGG Swiss water bottles cost about seventeen dollars for the smaller size, twenty-four dollars for the larger, but they last forever, never leach any bisphenol-A, and keep all those plastic bottles out of the landfill (plus my Mina swears they make her filtered tap water taste amazing!). ThinkSport also makes a safe steel bottle and it has an easy-to-carry sports handle. Finally sporty fave Nalgene has promised to switch to phthalate-free bottles by the end of 2008, but better toss your old ones, because many are leaching.

Wrap-N-Mat is an environmentally friendly sandwich wrap and place mat in one. It can be wiped or washed clean and used again and again. Good-bye to sticky, stinky petroleum-derived cling wraps and plastic bags. Plus they are waterproof and fabric, so you don't need to use all those paper towels. (Check out wrap-n-mat.com.)

YOU GOTTA THINK

My middle daughter used to just adore Barney. He's big, plush, and purple, and he sang to boot. What's not to love? (OK, I didn't love him, either, but welcome to parenthood.) Barney (energetically accompanied by my little Mina) loved to sing "I like to eat, eat, eat apples and bananas" over and over. But in reality, most kids do not like to eat, eat, eat apples and bananas or any kind of unadulterated fruits or veggies. They like to eat, eat, eat a lot of junk, and they like to throw, throw, throw the rest away!

According to a study reported on www.foodnavigator.com (Aug. 9, 2007), more and more parents are sending kids to school with healthy snacks, but up to seventy percent of children throw them away. The same survey found that ninety-seven percent of mothers want their children to eat nutritious snacks, whereas fifty-four percent of children want snacks that are tasty and sweet.

Why is it such a battle to serve up the good stuff to our families and in particular to our kids?

Well, here are just a few reasons:

• Ninety percent of foods marketed each year are processed foods.

• The food industry spends over thirty billion dollars a year marketing their products.

• Over thirty percent or ten billion dollars of that is spent marketing to children.

• In the last twelve months, about three thousand new desserts, cookies, candies, and snacks have been launched into the marketplace (and our children's consciousness). And they are all out to make a buck, or two, and most are very much directed at the demographic called KIDS.

So here's one way to save the day and have the snack actually end up in your kid's mouth instead of the garbage. Yes, after an intensive taste test, the Fassa girls are happy to share with you their list of the yummiest and (shh) healthiest energy bars around:

- Think energy bar (the Think5 is our fave)

- 365 Organic Everyday Value Honey Roasted Nut Bar

- Luna

- Clif Bar (Brownie is our favorite flavor)

The most important trick is to always have good, healthful snacks on hand. Let's face it: If it's hard to eat healthy, kids won't do it. Make it easy for your kids to make the smart choice. Try these other ideas for healthy snacks:

- Organic baby carrots in a bowl of water

- Washed organic fruit

- Stonyfield Farm organic yogurt smoothies

- Organic popcorn (and of course organic butter to go on top!)

HOW DOES YOUR GARDEN GROW?
One way to skip making your kids food? Have the school grow it! OK, not really *all* of it, but there is a great movement toward entire schools building gardening into the curriculum, and with good reason. After a lifetime of kids thinking food comes from boxes or cans, or wrapped in plastic, it's a real brain builder to actually experience that it all comes from the earth.

Again from our friends at BetterSchoolFood.org, check out the top ten reasons why gardens are a great idea.

1. Magic happens when a child harvests a vegetable he or she has planted and nurtured. The child will want to eat it!

It will increase interest and improve attitudes toward eating fruits and vegetables.

2. Students will learn where food really comes from—a carrot grows in the ground, a green bean on a vine and Brussels sprouts on a stalk!

3. School gardens foster an increased awareness of environmental issues. They will learn to respect and care for the soil, where our food comes from.

4. They will get to share their bounty with their classmates. Eating with their peers is one of the most important motivators for children to try new foods.

5. It gives children an opportunity to be outside and away from computer screens and, at the same time, significantly increase science achievement scores.

6. Gardening improves self-esteem, behavior, social skills, and interpersonal relationships as well as helps develop life skills including working with groups.

7. Research by Columbia Teachers College shows that hands-on gardening and cooking programs are the two things that are actually effective in behavior change; they get kids to eat more vegetables.

8. The gardens are beautiful spaces that connect students to their school and help them develop a sense of pride and ownership, which in turn improves attitudes toward school and discourages vandalism.

9. They provide opportunities for community involvement including neighbors, volunteers, parents, and local businesses.

10. School gardens promote good nutrition and exercise. The health of our kids and the health of our planet are fundamentally connected.

CONSCIOUS CONSUMERISM AND THE SEEMINGLY RELUCTANT TEEN

It may be possible to keep young kids focused on doing the right thing for themselves. I've had tremendous success in school (not me personally . . . former model, remember?) with my supersmart kids. I'm extremely lucky; I am the mom who goes to Back to School nights and gets firm handshakes and positive talk about high aptitude and performance. And believe me, I love it. But I'm gonna fess up—it's not always easy, mostly because they get to a certain age, and frankly, they get to make up their own mind. So we want to give our kids some strategies, and have some of our own, to help them stay on the healthy straight and narrow.

Here are my top four (and number five can be either pray or wish, depending on your belief system):

1. Help your kid understand the lesser of two evils, say the difference between choosing plain tortilla chips like Fritos and the MSG-flavored ones, Doritos.

2. Let your kids know that you understand that ultimately they are in charge of what goes into their mouths, but you don't plan to fund it if it's not fairly healthy.

3. Try to always have healthy food choices in nosh-sized portions available in the fridge and the cupboard. Teens do need a lot of food and when they need it, they need it NOW!

4. Finally, don't give up talking, even if you get rolling eyes and sighs. I have occasionally heard my ultracool teenage daughter talking about social responsibility, environmental justice, and organic agriculture to her posse of supersmart but seemingly sullen pals. And they're interested! Why not? They've got the big inheritance coming: the earth.

GREEN AT A GLANCE

Evergreen: Take on the school food mafia. Form a wellness committee and ask to review everything from ingredients to the shelf time for canned goods.

Pea green: Be vigilant about making your kids' lunches and choose responsibly about how you send them.

Spring green: Talk—and listen—to your kids about what they think about the environment, food, and the rest of the world!

Part III

A World
of Good

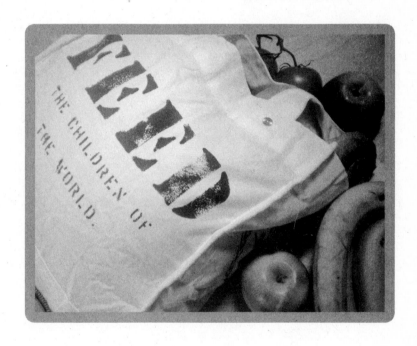

*The Toughest Job
You'll Ever Love—
Welcome to Parenthood*

One Big ~~Hippie~~ Happy Family

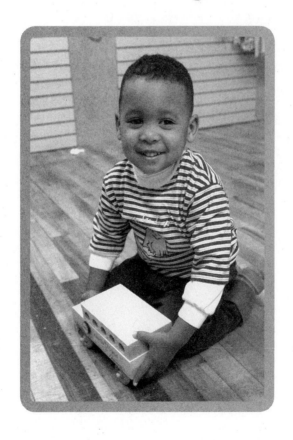

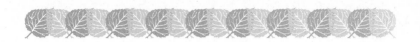

Totally Unplugged, or
How to Reconnect
When You Disconnect

You can have it all: one big happy family. OK, I don't know about the big part—that's up to you and your mate. But you can be happy. Not in that weird, perfect Stepford Wife way, and you also don't need to sequester your brood in some *Little House on the Prairie* remote landscape. But, with a little soul-searching and focus, you can find your family's own resonating, memorable, unique togetherness style. It doesn't need to cost much—in fact, it's often the free things that help us have the best times of our lives. This chapter is all about the fun family stuff that you can do with your critters. Cool, healthy, green, and off-the-grid stuff. Because the family that plays together stays together. Birds of a feather flock together. Take a hike, ride your bike. Family game nights avoid many fights. OK, I'll spare you any more of my poetry (but, hey, that's a good, wholesome pastime for you and your kids, too: brainteasers and rhyme time!).

If you really don't do much *en famille* except plop on the sofa and watch the tube, you'll want to start out slowly, like you did with family dinners. I'd suggest a mandatory unplugged family game night. (You can introduce electronic fun like a movie or the Wii later, when you're enjoying more than one night a week together.) Choose an area—if you don't have a rec room, the kitchen or dining room table is fine—and bring out the games. Keep a selection of tried-and-true people pleasers on hand. Here are some of our favorites:

- Deck of cards

- Clue

- Apples to Apples

- Game of Life

- Sequence

- Guess Who?

- Checkers

- Chess

- Scrabble

If you don't already have a good stock of games, these are well worth the outlay of cash for the hours and hours of fun you can get out of them. They're all widely available online and in stores. However, if you're in a green recycling mode (and also want to hold on to some green), you can pick up awesome bargains at yard sales or Web sites like Freecycle.org and Craigslist.org.

Keep in mind that younger kids in particular will be more engaged if the games you choose are noncompetitive or lightly competitive. Cranium makes great innovative board games that fit the bill, like Cadoo and Whoonu. And charades has a place for everyone and is worth making a family tradition.

Even deciding who picks the game can be fun. Roll the dice, or if you're active, consider a quick game of musical chairs: The last one sitting chooses the first game. So everyone has a chance, though, have the player to the left choose the next game.

Totally homemade versions might fit your family. A hum-along version of *Name That Tune* can turn into your own hilarious version of *America's Funniest Home Videos.* And I'll tell you, it's actually a lot more fun to be looking at your family and laughing than laughing at someone else's family on the small screen. So go for it, and just ignore those teenagers' slumped shoulders; they'll have a great time soon enough, too.

PITCH IN AND PICK UP

Do your kids have the sense that your home is theirs in terms of inviting friends for sleepovers or leaving their school supplies in every imaginable area, but maybe not so much when it comes to raking the leaves or straightening up their rooms?

If your kids are dutifully finishing their homework so they can rush downstairs to help you set the dinner table, or fighting over who can wash and fold that huge pile of laundry, you can feel free to skip this part. But if, like most of us, you often just cave and do all the dirty work yourself because it seems like so much more trouble to get them to do it, you may want to rethink and revamp your approach. You'll be much happier and have a lot more time to do fun family stuff together if you can get your kids to pitch in more around the house. It builds responsibility, and even though they may groan at first, it makes for a stronger, more balanced family. Here are some strategies that may help you implement this:

• Take some time with your mate to decide what you think are reasonable expectations of everyone (not just the kids). Then have a family meeting and let the kids know you value their contributions and want to improve fill-in-the-blank (the house, the backyard, your bank account, etc.). If you can include your kids in the discussion of who does which specific chores and when, they are more likely to join your team and benefit greatly from feeling needed (as opposed to forced into service).

• Pop a chart on the fridge. If you've got one of those glamorous steel ones that won't take magnets, consider a dry-erase board hung in a prominent place, such as over the breakfast table.

• Being somewhat flexible can increase cooperation. Let the kids occasionally trade duties or days.

Pretty soon it should be a habit, and you'll all have more downtime to spend together, too.

TOYLAND
The entertainment landscape our kids face today has changed so much from when we were kids, or even waaaaayyyyyy back when our parents were tykes. Toys in particular have changed. What are now called interactive toys are not really so interactive at all. A walking, talking, remote-controlled robot does not engage a child in the same way that a wooden train set does. Plastic toys may be

colorful and engaging, but most of them also contain phthalates, industrial chemicals that can leach into a child's bloodstream and have significant health effects. And as all the scary recalls have shown us, we have to look out for toxins like lead paint.

What makes the biggest difference between kids who are on a happy quest for learning and those who flounder? There is a strong connection between what our kids play with and the creation of who they are and the life we want for them, on two levels.

First, of course we want the best for our children, and therefore we're probably going to screen out violent video games that show blow-'em-up school buses and the like (no, I'm not kidding). Second, we want to be sure the playthings they have in such close proximity are benign and safe in their components and chemical makeup.

The first of these is probably easier to enforce because, thank goodness, there are federal guidelines to follow (however general) that can help us ascertain the age appropriateness of the game. But determining the actual physical safety of our kids' playthings is not so easy or clear. We seem to live in a recall world, where "better safe than sorry" has hardly been heard. We need to be vigilant; if it seems too good to be true—i.e., the toys have too-bright colors, are too inexpensive, have a questionable country of origin—we need to ask ourselves if the potential downside, including toxins, developmental delays, and dangerous recalls, is part of what we're buying into. We have control over what goes into our shopping carts and into our kids' hands.

There are some people who have such a strong sense of self that when they have kids, they really become Jung's archetype of the consummate Earth Mother (or the intuitive Primitive Man), mashing organic sweet potatoes and screening every possible toxin from their children's reach. My green light turned on when

I had my first, but it took me years to figure out how to explain, with perseverance and a polite smile, that I wanted extended-family members to respect my green choices for my kids. If only I had known Tricia McElwee back then, then maybe my husband's aunt would still be talking to me.

Green Guru

Tricia McElwee

ONE HUNDRED PERCENT NATURAL MOM

Meet a green vigilante who knows how to have her organic cake and let others enjoy their choices, too, all while protecting her little ones from all kinds of harm.

"We like to keep the media out of our house—we have a TV, but it's behind doors, and we make an effort to watch only after our two-year-old has gone to bed. We let her watch some of the fun specials—we enjoyed *Rudolph* when we were little, so we want her to have the same experience— but not every day.

"I only purchase natural toys. We always choose hand-made and wooden or natural fabric. We want to cultivate more creative play versus the toy being the thing. And the natural toys are made really well, so they'll last longer; they'll make it through more kids whether you have more or donate to another family. You'll be able to pass down a great toy from generation to generation.

"We also want to avoid plastics because of the PVCs,

phthalates, and other toxins. They have been proven to cause developmental delays and birth defects. Plus, these same poisons are contaminating the planet where they're made—who wants to be part of that?

"The toy industry is not well regulated, and until it is, we, as parents, need to take responsibility for what is in their little lives. As sad as all the recalls are, now the cat is out of the bag—we all know we need to be more careful. The Environmental Working Group is a great resource for safe products and toys. (See www.ewg.org.)

"Of course my loving family wants to get our daughter lots of what they consider fun toys, but I tell them honestly that if they send us something that is not appropriate, we'll just donate it. Since they don't want to waste their money, they do get the ones we want. Whenever I e-mail suggestions of what to get her for her birthday or Christmas, I list the reasons we have our restrictions, so they have a better understanding of why we're asking what we are.

"As a parent, I can't just pass the buck. It's my job to choose what my kids have access to."

Red Flag

Skip bargain toys from the dollar store or any other hard-to-track deep discounter.

Avoid plastics, especially squishy plastics. They have a high likelihood of being made of polyvinyl chloride (PVC) and may even be fixed with lead.

Take a pass on the "does everything under the sun" toy that also "takes two nine-volt batteries." Over the lifetime of the toy, you'll probably spend many times the original cost of the toy on replacement batteries (and the sounds and lights may also drive you nuts!).

Green Flag

Check out a huge selection of wooden toys, from little figurines to swanky dollhouses, at the appropriately named www.wooden toys.com.

Earth to Kid, our own simple small line of U.S.-made heirloom-quality toys, is made from sustainably managed forests (www.earthtokid.com).

Toys "R" Us now has a terrific line called Good Green Fun that is smooth, Forest Stewardship Council certified (FSC), and built to build growing imaginations. No paint, so none of those scary recall issues. Available at all Toys "R" Us locations or online at www.toysrus.com.

Melissa & Doug makes toys that are really reasonably priced, and good quality for the price. They're not FSC certified but always better than plastic (www.melissaanddoug.com).

YOU CAN DO IT—DO IT YOURSELF!

Sometimes you don't even need to buy any toys. As every parent knows, there's a reason for the cliché of your kid liking the box the gift came in more than the gift itself. More often than not, it's hilariously true. Here's a Green Guru with the experience and know-how to help you get your green groove on with your kid. Cost? Zero dollars.

Green Guru

Dr. Lisa Ecklund-Flores

NEONATAL DEVELOPMENTAL PSYCHOLOGIST

FOUNDER AND DIRECTOR, CHURCH STREET SCHOOL

FOR MUSIC AND ART, MANHATTAN

PROFESSOR, MERCY COLLEGE

MOM

Dr. Ecklund-Flores is a developmental psychologist specializing in early-childhood experience. Her Church Street School is a community school, but as I have learned from Dr. Ecklund-Flores, community is really just a bunch of individuals living in the same place with some of the same wants, needs, desires, and dreams. Looking at it that way, the whole world is our community . . . and on a very practical level, you can make the world a better place by the things you do with your own kids, in your own home. You'll have the time of your life, and it won't cost you a cent.

"Children learn by running, jumping, singing, and clapping. Every one of us is a unique constellation of passions and skills, and I think it's our job as parents to support and guide our children in this journey—to help them find their creative voices. Since music and art are nonverbal and fundamentally physical, there is little to limit kids' creative expression.

"There are three organic approaches that help kids attain a healthy sense of self. We base our programs around them at my school, but you can do them at home, too."

Music

When looking for music classes for your children, look for teachers who can harness your child's physical energy and channel it into activities that require ear, mind, and body to work together in an upbeat and fun-loving way.

You Can Do It, Too

Make beautiful music at home! Try these simple activities.

• **Dance.** Hold your toddler in your arms and dance to music of different styles so he can feel the difference in the rhythm and tempo with his whole body. Be responsive to the music—stop moving during breaks in the song; spin around on the accents. Break out some of your all-time favorite CDs and dance away!

• **Make a band.** Tap on a drum or shake bells with your toddler to recorded music of different styles and speeds. Remember, try to be responsive to changes in the music when you're playing. This will promote the development of sensorimotor coordination in your child.

• **Play duets.** Sit with your preschooler at a piano or keyboard and play echo games. Play a brief combination of notes or rhythms and have your child play them back to you. Start simply with one or two notes and work up from there. Be playful, take turns!

• **Make a musical.** Invent or read a story or poem with your preschooler and use the piano or other instruments to create the "soundtrack." Create the sound of rainstorms, or flowers growing. Record your performance for posterity!

• **Quick reaction.** Stopping-and-starting games are great fun for kids, too. Freeze Dance is a popular version of this (or old-fashioned musical chairs). Anticipating rests in music and responding with the whole body is another fun way to build coordination.

• When your child reaches the appropriate age (six to twelve years) to begin instrumental-music lessons, find a teacher who includes improvisation and composition as part of the lesson routine, in addition to note reading. Both improvisation and composition connect the player with the instrument directly, allowing him to express himself in his own unique way.

Art
The arts can help children feel confident and competent and give them a forum to exercise their creativity. Making art helps develop their minds and their self-esteem at the same time. Choose an art class for your child that uses great materials and open-ended projects—projects whose outcome is defined by your child. Techniques should be offered in an unstructured way rather than teaching how to create art that "looks like" something.

You Can Do It, Too
Lots of parents stay away from art projects at home because of the messiness factor. But it's actually really important that kids don't get hung up about the mess when making

art, or they will be too concerned about getting their hands dirty to ever truly explore their creativity. Try these time-tested art projects.

• Toddlers like to poke their fingers in homemade play dough (two parts flour, one part salt; add water until the desired consistency, and knead!). When they've exhausted the possibilities of shapes and prints they can make with their hands, they can use spoons, forks, and cups. Pasta of different sizes can be pushed into the dough to make works of art, too.

• Fruit and vegetable prints are a fun project for preschoolers because they're almost instantaneous. Apples, oranges, and peppers are great choices; cut the fruits or vegetables in half so that your child can see the different patterns and textures. Then you and your child can easily create beautiful prints when you dip them into a thin layer of paint and press them on a piece of paper. Experiment with tempera paint of different colors and various sizes and textures of paper for different effects.

• Kids of all ages like to drip small amounts of paint on paper and fold the paper in half to create an "inkblot." Each time you unfold your paper, you reveal a one-of-a-kind abstract work of art. Create a series for your home art gallery!

• Your elementary-school-aged kids will enjoy making a life-sized self-portrait. Have them lie down on a large sheet of butcher paper or recycled mural paper. Trace their body with a marker. Then they can spend the rest of the afternoon creating their self-portrait, using yarn or shredded paper for hair, fabric for clothes, markers to draw their facial expression, and so on. Their artwork can become the newest and coolest poster in their room. Developing self-image is huge for kids at this age, so the project will be both art and therapy at the same time!

Let Them Follow Their Bliss

No matter what activities your child is engaged in, allow her to express her independence, competence, and skills whenever possible. This means inside the home as well as out; parents can have a huge impact by carefully choosing the child's academic and extracurricular activities to promote the sensibilities that are developmentally appropriate, and by incorporating those same sensibilities at home. (Don't try to push children ahead—it doesn't make them smarter, and it can burn them out.)

You Can Do It, Too

When you engage in music and art activities at home, let your kids take the lead.

• Let toddlers choose what instruments you'll play, the kind of music you'll listen to, the color paint you'll use, and where you'll put the prints on the paper.

• Use a portable CD player that your preschooler can operate himself. Let your child put the instruments away. Help her make the play dough herself!

> • Be sure extracurricular activities are not overly focused on competition and performance, and look for cooperative experiences, too, such as partner lessons on an instrument, group drum circles, or collaborative mural projects.

IT'S WHICH CRAFT?

Another great thing to do with your kids is crafting. And sometimes, it feels like a real lifesaver. It is a way to be together yet experience the solitude of art, all without worrying too much about rigid process or perfect results. One of our favorite crafts came out of pure necessity: about a gajillion bored kids. Here's how it happened.

On a cold winter's day, in a deep and dark December, the phone call came early, breaking the eerie morning calm and dragging me out of my cozy bed. With foreboding I picked up the receiver. An inhuman voice spoke the words I had come to dread: "This is the public school system. Due to inclement weather, school will be closed today." Nooooooo!

This parental horror was followed by a series of rants, raves, and relentless begging from employed friends who needed a place to park their kids for the day. First cheerfully, then begrudgingly, I offered sanctuary for their little ones, thinking it would be an easy day of snowball fights in the backyard followed by blanket forts and hot cocoa in the playroom.

But the winds were not with me that day (or shall I say the rains). Instead of snowman-friendly flakes, we got torrential sleet and hail. And there I was with eight kids, counting my own, at the kitchen table. Well, necessity really is the mother of invention. I hauled out the organic-cotton scraps my husband refused to toss from our Green Babies cuttings and got crafty.

Making Organic-Cotton Rag Dolls

You may not have organic cotton at home, but you can still create your own sustainable soft buddy by recycling a favorite T-shirt into a work of folk art.

What You'll Need
old T-shirt for cutting
scissors
cotton string
various printed jersey fabrics
permanent markers
craft glue

Directions

1. Start with a piece of stretchy jersey cotton fabric (like T-shirt fabric). You want a piece that is about 10 × 10 inches. Using soft scraps to stuff the "head," make a "ghost" by tying string around the neck.

2. Tie off 2 points about 1 inch above the bottom corners for the feet.

3. Cut a piece of fabric (same color as ghost) about 5 × 2 inches and twist it into a rope to tie around the waist. Now tie off the 2 corners above it with string, about 1 inch from edges, to make hands.

4. Choose colorful fabrics you love for the clothes. Cut out a rectangle and then cut a slit in the center. Slip it over your

doll's head. Create a skirt by pulling the fabric down to the waist and tying with string, or a dress by tying a belt. A poncho can top it off with no extra tie.

5. Next, decorate your doll's face with your permanent markers. Be creative and let the doll express how you feel!

6. Your doll is ready for its hair. Usually it's best to use a solid-colored piece of fabric, about 2½×3½ inches for long hair or 2½×1 inch for short hair. Cut ¼-inch fringe on both sides for bangs and back of hair.

7. Generously apply craft glue directly to the hair and gently put it on the doll's head. Press firmly with the palm of your hand while you concentrate on what you want to name your new friend.

▶ You are done! You have turned something old into something beautiful, an original piece of folk art!

TREASURE OUT OF TRASH

There are certain things you probably have "around" when you have a family. You know what I mean: super-ugly luggage that doesn't match (but that you're sure you might need someday), puffy coats and clunky rain boots (because Mother Nature can be a mutha), hideous hand-me-downs for the kids from well-meaning friends that never seem to fit but that you are reluctant to pass on "just in case."

All right, if none of that describes you and you think you've escaped membership in the aforementioned club, check this: Bet you've got mismatched pillowcases and loads of lonely single socks. Never fear, I've got the domestic diva, the magical maven, the woman who can help you turn your nagging clutter into works of art. Meet Jasmin, the Worsted Witch. Check out her site to help you conjure up your own treats, or great crafted gifts.

Green Guru

Jasmin Malik Chua
WRITER, TREEHUGGER.COM, PLANETGREEN.COM
FOUNDER, WORSTEDWITCH.COM

There's a movement going on: Everyone you know is into knitting, scrapbooking, rejuvenating old frames and knick-knacks. What's so great about these old-fashioned pastimes? They're good for the earth—but they're good for you, too. They relax the mind, provide a creative outlet, occupy our kids, and give us something beautiful to look at or give to someone else. Jasmin knows this, and knows it so well, she can help us all learn to craft sustainably.

"I'm a knitter, so it started because I was looking for yarns I could use that were sustainable rather than synthetic. But my idea of sustainability morphed into all kinds of crafts people can do to help the environment. Realistic, meaningful, yet easy things they can do without sacrificing their way of life.

"I'm a terrible pack rat, so I save buttons, bits of ribbon, and colored tissue paper, and I always keep interesting jars. When I want to make homemade gifts, I already have what I need.

"There's no such thing as a useless item. You can fill up an orphan sock with some buckwheat and a couple of pinches of organic lavender, and sew up the opening. Nuke the sock for a couple of minutes in the microwave for an instant hand warmer, or use it as is for a wrist rest when you're working on the computer. Out of an old pillowcase, make a simple drawstring laundry or overnight bag. Cut two two-inch slits on the open side of the pillowcase (use the seams as a guide). Next, fold down the fabric inward and sew along the horizontal edges. Insert a long piece of ribbon through this new casing to act as your drawstring. Voilà!"

Relaxing Lavender Bath Salts

coarse sea salt
Epsom salts
lavender essential oil
geranium essential oil
dried organic lavender
clean, empty jars
spice sachets (or unbleached cheesecloth)

▶ *Cost: a couple of dollars at most per jar, compared with more than $20 at a bath and body store.*

1. Combine 3 cups of salt with 1 cup of Epsom salts in a clean bowl. Add 4–5 drops of each oil.
2. Sprinkle in a pinch or 2 of dried lavender. Mix well.
3. Pour into jars.
4. Decorate the jars as fancily as you desire.
5. Include some premade spice sachets or cotton tea bags with your gift, for holding the salts when used in the bathtub

(they corral floating herbs, so the bather gets the aromatic benefits without having to pick the bits out after the soak). Alternatively, cut a circle measuring at least 8 inches in diameter out of unbleached cheesecloth, and instruct your gift recipient to scoop some bath salts in the middle, then gather up the edges of the cheesecloth into a knot.

Bittersweet Chocolate and Orange Lip Balm
MAKES 1 SMALL CONTAINER.

▶ *Shelf life: around 4 months.*

3 tablespoons organic cocoa butter
3–4 organic, fair trade dark chocolate chips
1 teaspoon vitamin E oil
1/4 teaspoon organic orange extract

1. Melt the cocoa butter in the microwave.
2. Add the chocolate chips and stir until melted. (You may have to microwave the mixture again for a few seconds.)
3. Add vitamin E (a natural preservative) and orange extract.
4. Mix well and pour into a small container.

GREEN AT A GLANCE

Evergreen: Have a craft corner. Keep little bits of "pretty things": interesting stamps off of mail, bits of ribbon, buttons, etc. You'll be ready for arts and crafts anytime.

Pea green: Make family game night a priority at least once a week, and consider making noncompetitive choices so everyone "wins."

Spring green: Remind yourself that the box is often better than the toy! Instead of taking your kid shopping for a toy, make your own fun together.

That's Entertainment

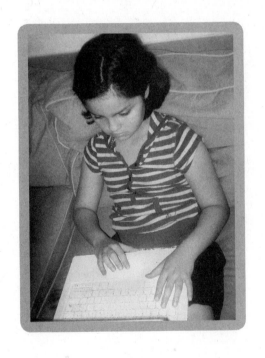

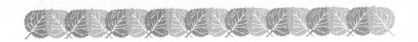

Tuned In and Connected

For most of us, a totally TV-free home is not very realistic, and perhaps not too appealing, either. I am right there with (most) of you. So carefully making the transition into welcoming that seductive colorful box is what this chapter is all about. Because you don't want to end up with a free-for-all gorge on 899 channels and a bunch of couch potato zombies, I'll offer you several different approaches to a green and modified TV (and computer) life.

Here's the abbreviated story of how it went for my family:

- *First kid: no TV in the house.*

- *Second kid: one TV but husband rigged it so we could get only PBS (except Sunday nights when we could switch to HBO for* Curb Your Enthusiasm*).*

- *Third kid: little TV that picked up only broadcast stations until the lumbering television antenna on the roof fell off in a windy storm. Practically overnight, that was replaced by cable, and every imaginable channel.*

That's actually what happened, and eventually it may happen to you, too. Here's the slightly longer version of my family's relationship with the magic box.

In the city we did opt for TV free, but that's easy when your child is under five and there are other like-minded folks to arrange playdates with. But as your kids grow, and mingle with others whose parents aren't Luddites, it becomes much, much harder to keep the outside world, well, out. Besides, there is something to be said for limited "exposure" and building immunity. Beyond missing the entertainment value (which, let's face it, can be high), completely banning TV can turn it into the coveted Golden Fleece, and instill it with a mystique and allure that would turn Svengali green (with envy, not the good green). So you may want to take it easy, be flexible, and open that Pandora's box just a little, while still keeping the plagues and pestilence to a minimum.

Below is our set of rules and you can take them, leave them, or adapt them to your own needs. With these, we have found great happiness with the magic box. . . .

FIVE RULES FOR TV SUCCESS

1. No TV after school or in the evening on school nights

2. Even on total veg-out days, no more than two hours unless there's a family show we all want to watch together

3. No R-rated movies (duh!)

4. When Mom or Dad says enough, no questions asked. (OK, this doesn't actually work nearly as well as planned.)

5. There are occasional exceptions to every rule (except the R-rating rule, which stays firmly in place).

If you need fortification to lock it down or just say no, remember:

ACCORDING TO THE AMERICAN ACADEMY OF PEDIATRICS

• The average child watches three hours of TV a day—two hours of quality programming is the maximum recommended by the academy.

• Active-play time is needed to develop mental, physical, and social skills.

• Children who watch violence on TV are more likely to display aggressive behavior.

• Young children don't know the difference between programs and commercials.

WATCH THIS

Keep in mind, though, sometimes judiciously choosing and watching a quality show on TV is actually as good as—and occasionally even better than—almost anything else. It can be as inspirational as a trip to a museum or even as meaningful as a good read. As a parent, one of the things I really want to do is to open doors for my kids, to kindle their imaginations. I'm a great believer in thoughtful daydreaming, and I try to lay out a smorgasbord for my kids so they can observe, consider, and pull out what fires them up.

My middle one, Mina, is a budding chef (a culinary genius!) and she really loves cooking shows. Because she's a vegetarian and a nature lover, her absolute favorite show is *Get Fresh with Sara Snow* on Discovery Health.

Green Guru

Sara Snow

HOST, *GET FRESH WITH SARA SNOW*

HEALTH DISCOVERY

Sara came into the green life a little differently than most of us did—most of us entered to improve our health and our lives, or to step up to our roles as responsible, loving parents. But Sara was born green. In fact, you might even call her a true Green Baby! Sara grew up in a Utopian natural family. Her mom and dad founded Eden Foods, one of the oldest and most credible natural-food companies on the planet. Her natural physical beauty and ease with people made her a magnet for TV, and she knew her message was easy and do-able enough for this influential, expansive medium.

"TV is the medium that has the ability to reach families, many families, where the desire to live healthy is so strong. I focus on food. Food is so important. We eat three times—or twenty times—every day! We are what we eat, so a huge number of our healthy lifestyle choices revolve around food. Healthy choices begin at home—fresh fruits, nutrient-rich vegetables instead of junk—but it's also about choosing local and organic whenever possible. Forge a relationship with farmers at your local market or farms in your CSA (Community-Supported Agriculture). You'll be getting fresh foods straight from the person who grew it. It's so important for kids to grow up understanding where food comes from: A farmer grew it. Picked it. Brought it.

"My mantra is 'Make the changes in the choices—and make better choices.' Green is good and happy and pretty and fun. Because I grew up in this world, and my family was part of it for so long, it's fun to see the whole rest of the world joining us. We're all connected!"

THE OTHER BOX WITH MORE THAN SIXTY-FOUR COLORS

Nope, I don't mean Crayola. When you have kids in the house, a computer is soon to follow. Eventually they'll need it to do their homework, and chances are, you'll occasionally want to Google something, as well. But because of the great access to information, both good and bad, that the computer provides, it becomes difficult to keep the genie in the bottle. I admit that this is an endless balancing act, but I have found you another powerful ally.

WII THE PEOPLE

After much discussion and research, we recently purchased a Wii game system for our TV. In case this phenomenon has escaped

Elisabeth Hickey
CHALLENGE/ENRICHMENT TEACHER
MOM OF THREE

She's an expert from the trenches: a mother of three and a challenge teacher of gifted and talented students in the public school system of Westchester County. Elisabeth Hickey has a few tricks for us about how to keep kids amused while developing their big gray muscle, and balancing in some realistic computer and TV time.

"None of my kids can watch TV, play video games, or play noneducational computer games during the week. It's pretty much zero, an absolute no, unless there is a special we all can enjoy together. On the weekends they can each have an hour a day of playing on the computer or vegging out in front of the TV. Sometimes on weekend nights we'll pool our time and watch a movie together.

"When my kids say, 'I'm bored,' I say, 'Go read—make something—play your music. . . .' That's how talents develop.

"When it comes to computer time, I agree that it is very tough to reel the kids in from all of this media. As they get older, the draw is too strong, particularly if they have a lot of friends or specific interests in things like sports and music. YouTube, although a great resource, can be a great time waster (and brain drainer), as well. The problem is, kids will hear about something at school that they want to watch, and come home to take a peek. Since a lot of that stuff is interesting and/or funny, as a parent I can get caught up in it, too. It's hard to say no, particularly if I find it fascinating, as well! If this happens to you, you may have to make a concerted effort to pull back and reinstate rules that may have slackened. When I do, I meet with some resistance, but I try not to cave and do my best to stand up for my principles. Most of the time it works, but not always.

"However, I think that the kids, down deep, appreciate the limits we put on them because freedom is a tough sentence for a child. As I tell my middle schooler, 'Just because you're getting older does not mean you get more freedom; it actually means you get less. You are entering the time of the "stupids" and it is my job to see you through them safely, with as few injuries as possible.' I don't always get a cheery smile from him in return, but I have gotten good at turning my back on him.

FAVORITE WEB SITES DIVIDED BY AGE

0–4 None. I don't think kids this young should be on the Internet.

5–8 www.webkinz.com
www.crickweb.co.uk

9–11 www.discovery.com
www.nationalgeographic.com

In every case, set time limits and cross your fingers!

FAVORITE BOARD GAMES

- Goblet

- Backgammon

- Senet

- Mancala

- Blokus

"These are all games that involve strategy, thought, and fine motor skills, but they're also a lot of fun. For one-person games I recommend Rush Hour and Hi-Q."

you, it's not your average video game system. Unlike most video games, Wii games are physically interactive; instead of punching buttons or keys, you have to move your body to play (e.g., swing your arm when you're playing tennis, bend your knees to turn on the ski slope, wave your arms to make Mario jump and spin in Super Mario Brothers). It also has hookups to kid faves like Guitar Hero, in which you can play Foghat's classic "Slow Ride" over and over and over on a toy guitar (but thankfully with modified lyrics). My very levelheaded friend Nichelle had this to say about her family and the Wii: "We limit TV to a half hour to an hour on Fridays and Sundays. On Saturdays Alexis sometimes whines and complains, but then she moves on, as it's not going to change the outcome. My partner and I had talked about getting the Wii, but it's very expensive. Then we realized it's not your typical video game system; if it's raining, we could still play tennis on the Wii—we could all play baseball. Now we also do karaoke or dance moves.

The other day I watched Alexis create a video on the Wii and I was blown away. Now she has confidence and she believes she can make a movie, and you know what? I do, too!"

IT'S SHOWTIME

My husband is a former theater director, and at one time worked with the Paper Bag Players, the renowned children's theater company. So he is pretty picky about what films our kids see. When he has his way, thank goodness, there is no *Grudge 2* for our teen, no *Porky's 4* for our tween, and definitely no *Bratz* for our grade-schooler.

So what's left?

Well, here's just a brief list of what I think are the most entertaining, age-appropriate, and possibly even brain-building films that are a decidedly deeper shade of green:

• *Pocahontas*: OK, it might not be historically accurate, but the message of Grandmother Willow is both memorable and awe-inspiring—plus Vanessa Williams belting out "Colors of the Wind" is enough to convert an Exxon executive!

• *The Simpsons Movie*: Not perfectly clean (big surprise), but as always, *The Simpsons* delivers a kindhearted critique, this time on one of the most profound issues of our time, our environment, and the all-too-human desire to slack off. Sharp and pretty funny, too.

• *When Tomorrow Comes*: a chilling but pretty convincing fairy tale about how little time we might have left to do right by Gaia, and a refreshing look at how connected we all are to one another.

• *March of the Penguins*: an irresistible tale of those adorable, indomitable creatures that also conveys a powerful message about the environment.

• *The Future of Food*: Watching this amazing doc is a way we can all understand, in about ninety minutes, how profoundly genetic engineering has altered what we eat. It's inspiring and entertaining.

• *An Inconvenient Truth*: My husband and I were invited to the New York premiere of Al Gore's now-famous film, and honestly, there were empty seats. Now, only a few short years later, it's one of the most celebrated films in my lifetime. Al Gore and the brave Laurie David, who made the film, have given our kids and grandkids an opportunity to thrive on a healthy planet, if we all heed their message, and act together, today.

• *Born Free*: This ancient pic still resonates with timely love between the human species and animals. Definitely inspiring.

A CRITICAL EYE

It's always a good idea to talk with your kids about the message behind the movie. Sometimes kids derive a different message from the one we expect! And definitely talk to them about marketing and branding. Megahits like *High School Musical* can be fun to do karaoke to, and may even have a positive message like "Be true to yourself," but do you really want to pop for the endless stream of *HSM* trinkets and tie-ins? If you take the time to teach your child to defend against this kind of marketing onslaught, not only will it be easier on your wallet, but your kids will be more discerning consumers for life—of films and everything else. At the same time, pics that don't have any of that slick marketing muscle can ultimately have the most impact on your child's worldview and morals, so it may be worth it to opt for the indie when possible.

AT THE MOVIES—ON A BUDGET? Perhaps you are short of cash . . . and frankly, who isn't these days? We love a great movie, but it costs a small fortune to take three kids and two adults out (and my kids frown on my old frugal habit of sneaking—ahem, augmenting—the popcorn supply by bringing our own—organic!— from home). So, it costs fifty to a hundred dollars to take the family to the movies—that's just not doable, at least not very often. The living room is a great alternative. You can have family movie night, like family game night, practically for free!

Here's one great help: BarterBee bills itself as "the cheapest way to trade movies, music and games," and besides your own relatives, they actually are. Here's how it works: Listing and sending off your used CDs and DVDs earns you points, which you can then use to purchase used media from other BarterBee.com members. (The number of points depends on the condition of what you're sending in.) This is not only, of course, a great way to save greenbacks, but a great way to be green, too: instant recycling. Check it out at www .barterbee.com.

GREEN AT A GLANCE

 Evergreen: Limit screen time. Choose only PBS or educational shows.

Pea green: Enlist everyone in a plan to choose TV you can all enjoy together, or invest in a Wii and make that part of your screen time.

Spring green: Put the computer in a family-friendly area so you have a good idea of the sites your kids are visiting and the amount of time they're spending online. Talk with your kids about advertising and how it works.

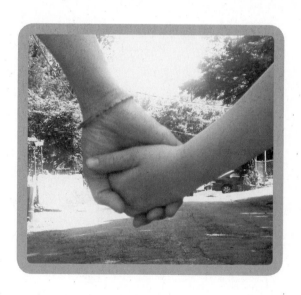

You Are the Change You Wish to See in the World

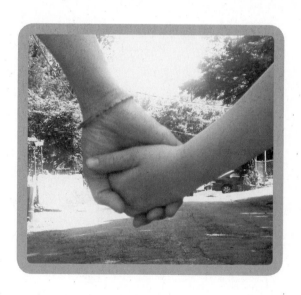

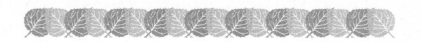

The Great Green Connectedness of Everything

I t takes a lot of cojones, to paraphrase Gandhi, to "be the change you wish to see in the world." But justice, equality, happiness, abundance, peace . . . they're all possible. Right now. No more wishing. It's within our reach, in this lifetime, and it can be our gift, the legacy we leave our kids. All we need to do is wake up, acknowledge our power, and recognize that we indeed are the change.

We are what we eat, wear, buy, and do. And our choices make all the difference in the world.

YOU ARE WHAT YOU EAT: *BON APPÉTIT*

In many ways, we are the luckiest of the lot, those of us with that little paunch, those extra five pounds, sweating through crunches and paying trainers to help us waddle off the weight. As you know, not everyone in the world has the luxury of easy access to lots of food. Trace any of our families just a few generations back, and chances are, the daily pursuit of enough to eat took up most of the day. Even though the majority of us still work hard to make the dough for our daily bread, things have changed, and they certainly have gotten a lot more comfortable. Here in the West, in four or five short generational blinks, we've leaped from going to bed with hunger pangs to waking up wondering how to lose that extra pad we've acquired on our belly and tush.

We humans are hardwired to love food, and when we have a VIP pass to the beautiful steel box in the kitchen day and night, it's no wonder we're carrying a little extra. But along with all this bounty, more choices at every meal than kings and queens had in times past, we've lost something. We've drifted far away from the true essence of food. With all our irradiating, shrink-wrapping, prewashing, and precutting, we've lost sight of a simple truth: Food comes from nature, and there is a symphony of rhythmic, natural, cyclical events that occur to bring forth the life that becomes our food, this food that so generously gives us life.

Green Guru

Lizanne Falsetto
FOUNDER, THINK ENERGY BARS
MOTHER OF TWO

When you see those gorgeous, super-fit people running around, sometimes with a gaggle of kids in tow and often with a dog to boot, do you ever wonder how they have so much health and vitality? I used to convince myself it was the super iced mocha lattes from Dunkin' Donuts, but then I realized I actually never felt very energetic after chugging mine. Anyway, then I met Lizanne Falsetto, entrepreneur and mother of two. Lizanne always gives me the impression she has the six arms of a Hindu goddess because she is so hands-on busy and accomplishes so much. Yet she also has a grounded depth and calm to her. Let's find out how she does it all.

"I started my business to be able to offer other mothers and other working people an on-the-go and healthy choice.

"As rich as we are, the human population is starving themselves of green food and proper nutrition. Fruits and vegetables are such a huge part of health and wellness and the very thing that most young children are lacking. I wanted to eat healthy, but I didn't always have time, so I made an energy bar to nosh on when I was really on the go, or to stick in my kids' lunch boxes for snack time. Who needs a sugary pick-me-up that's going to knock you back down in twenty minutes?

"Fighting disease requires a strong immune system and that starts with a healthy diet. Today we have all these imbalances, a huge influx of poisons and toxins like never before. Food is the key to help our children and ourselves get healthy.

"Plus, organic food just plain tastes better than nonorganic. Compare an organic strawberry to a nonorganic one any day and I guarantee you'll taste the difference.

"I know it's more expensive. If you can't afford to buy organic all the time, pick the key items your family eats the most of—for example, milk, bread, apples, bananas, your favorite green leafy veggies, salad mix, or spinach.

"Healthy eating doesn't have to be a chore for you or your kids. If you make it fun for them, they'll eat it. Food is a fun activity. Every day I put out a big plate of veggies and ranch dip and let my kids play with the food as they eat. Who cares if they wear the olives on their fingers before they eat them?!"

Green Guru

Dr. Susan Rubin

FOOD EDUCATOR

FOUNDER, BETTER SCHOOL FOOD

MOM OF THREE

RETIRED DENTIST

All over the natural-products world I have met inspiring people, most often inspiring women. Women who are mothers and who, like me, had their green lights turn on because of the profound love—and lifestyle change—that motherhood brings. One of the most active, vocal, and informed women I've ever met is consumed with the desire to make life better for her kids, and for yours and mine, too. Meet the amazing Dr. Susan Rubin.

"One day twelve years ago my life changed. My five-year-old daughter came home from school with a backpack full of candy. I was a dentist, and I was incensed because of the possibility of tooth decay. How could my school be doling out candy when I was working so hard for health in my home? Eventually I ended up leaving my job and going back to school to become a nutritionist. Now I know that sugar does a lot more than damage teeth. Sugar acts like termites on the framework of our health. It just eats away at our solid foundations. Everyone thinks about sugar as a cause of obesity, but sugar also has a huge impact on behavior problems, asthma, and allergies. All these are connected to our overpackaged, overprocessed foods, and pound per pound, kids are infinitely more susceptible than adults. Poor-quality food is the basis of all these problems. That's why when babies have eczema, they can be cured through diet, or when kids have sinus and ear infections, eliminating dairy works so well.

"Eating is the most important thing we do every day and the easiest to control. We have free choice as to what we put in our shopping carts. Our three-year-olds aren't driving to the store."

SUSAN'S SEVEN STEPS FOR HEALTHIER KIDS

1. Walk your talk! It all starts with you. Set a good example. Your actions have a powerful impact on what your kids do. Work on yourself first; your kids will follow you.

2. The eighty/twenty rule: Strive to eat local, seasonal, organic, wholesome foods eighty percent of the time and don't feel guilty about the other twenty percent.

3. Don't bribe or reward kids with sugar or treats. Our kids need our time, love, and attention, not sugar! It's important to show our kids how to satisfy their emotional needs without food or material things.

4. Have healthy snacks readily available. Especially in the late afternoon. Fresh fruits and veggies are super easy—no packaged, processed, chemicalized food products necessary.

5. Involve your kids with shopping and preparing meals. This gives them a greater connection to, and appreciation for, food and where it comes from, and will make your life easier. Bring them to the farmers' market—you can't go wrong there!

6. Plant a garden. Growing food teaches on many levels. This is the most effective step you can take for better food and better health for your family and the planet. Easier on your wallet, too. Kids love eating the food they grew themselves.

7. Think of sleep as an important nutrient. Make sure everyone in your family gets enough sleep. Set solid rules on lights out.

Susan's Super-Easy Roasted Veggies

veggies (choose any of these: sweet potatoes, Yukon Gold potatoes, carrots, parsnips, cauliflower, green beans, Brussels sprouts, shallots)

olive oil
sea salt
any other spice such as garlic, rosemary, oregano, etc.

Cut veggies into bite-sized pieces. Mix and match and have fun!

Toss in a bowl with olive oil, sea salt, and spices.

Arrange veggies in single layer on baking sheet or roasting pan.

Place in oven.

Veggies are done when they are light brown, slightly crispy on the outside, and soft and sweet on the inside. Twenty minutes at 400–450 degrees is ideal for quick roasting that will ensure caramelized, crispy exteriors, but 325–350 will also work (if you've got other things in the oven that need a lower temperature). It just takes a bit longer.

Ovens vary, so check on veggies every 10 minutes. Give them a little shake in their tray and check if they're golden brown to see if they are done.

YOU ARE WHAT YOU WEAR:
YOU LOOK MARVELOUS

We humans have an incredibly intimate and loving relationship with what we wear. Our clothes warm us, protect us, and help us express who we are. If clothes make the man, they're also the architecture that holds together entire social systems. Clothing gets us noticed, and gets our kids accolades, too. And in case you are feeling a tad guilty about your bulging closets, remember: From the posh executive suite at Ralph Lauren to the hemp farms in rural China, the clothing you purchase provides jobs for hundreds of millions of people worldwide. So baby's adorable birthday suit is in a category of its own, but clothing is not a bad thing.

I've spent my entire adult life selling clothing in one incarnation or another: first modeling some of the most fabulous and expensive clothes in the world (alas, no, the model does not get to keep the clothes) and then founding and designing Green Babies, the world's oldest existing organic-cotton clothing company. I started Green Babies because

1. I needed a job (lots of extra baby weight made modeling in New York out of the question)

2. one of the only things I knew a lot about was clothing

3. I discovered—quite by chance—how devastating to our health and well-being conventional cotton is, and I thought I could make things a little better, one cute baby outfit at a time. (Plus my kid would be the best dressed on the playground!)

DID YOU KNOW?

• Cotton is the second-most-pesticide-laden crop in the world, after coffee, and number one in America.

• Conventional cotton occupies three percent of the world's farmland, but uses twenty-five percent of the earth's chemical pesticides and fertilizers.

• More energy is now used to produce synthetic fertilizers than to till, cultivate, and harvest all the crops in the U.S.

- Think you don't eat it? Check out your potato chips, cheese curls, corn chips. What's that near the top of the ingredients list? Yup, cottonseed oil.

My dream came true, thanks to people like you and other parents, grandparents, aunts, uncles, friends, and well-wishers who chose an organic-cotton garment to welcome a little one over a conventional-cotton one. I know for sure that what our kids wear affects our world, in so many matters-to-you ways. If you want to really do no harm, choose organic, buy "vintage" (thrift store), or choose something that benefits someone else directly, like TOMS Shoes. . . .

Green Guru

Blake Mycoskie
FOUNDER, TOMS SHOES

Sometimes the strangest things lead to greatness. My friend Brad introduced me to Blake, a visionary who took his love of life and fashioned it into a better way for others, namely, thousands of the world's poorest children. Sometimes, it's hard to believe how important a simple pair of shoes can be.

"In the wealthy first world, we have shoes to go to work in, shoes to run in, shoes to wear around the house, shoes to match our favorite outfits, and countless other pairs that we buy on a whim and then relegate to the back of our closets.

"My sister, Paige, and I competed on *The Amazing Race*. We spent thirty-one days begging and borrowing, chasing clues, and pretty much running constantly to try and win a one-million-dollar grand prize. My sister still gives me a hard time about botching our chances, but no matter. Had we won that prize, I almost certainly would not be where I am today, putting shoes on kids' feet and having the time of my life.

"This is what happened. After I finished *The Amazing Race*, I promised myself that I would return to all the mind-blowing places that we had blurred through. I went to South Africa, Belize, and finally Brazil and Argentina. About the last thing on my mind was starting a business. I planned on learning to sail, and playing some polo, and maybe having a few too many glasses of wine. Argentina is such an amazing place: beautiful, full of color, bustling with life, and, in pockets, heartbreakingly poor.

"Kids ran alongside the road, playing soccer and fetching water. But so few kids had the simple luxury of shoes. They'd develop cuts and scrapes on their feet, gnarly stuff that can lead to infections.

"At the same time, I discovered a kind of shoe called the alpargata that local farmers have been wearing for the past hundred years. It's as simple as a shoe can be, canvas up top and rope on the bottom. The guys that I was playing polo with had these shoes, as well as their girlfriends or wives. I bought a few pairs from local peddlers, and I too fell in love. I was wearing my alpargatas all of the time.

"So I had a wild idea. What if I created a company where for every pair of shoes I sold, I gave one away?

"In the past two years, TOMS has given away ten thousand pairs of shoes in Argentina and, most recently, fifty thousand pairs of shoes in South Africa. Sixty thousand pairs of shoes. A dream come true.

"The most amazing part of this story is that *individuals* have made this happen. An overwhelming number of TOMS sales come in orders of one and two pairs from people from all walks of life—Orange County surfer/skaters, fashionistas in New York City, soccer moms from the Midwest—pretty much the oddest collection of people you can think of.

"It doesn't matter who you are, or what you do, or how much money you have; *everyone* can make a difference. As consumers, we have great power. The companies that sell us shoes, and pants, and vegetables, and toilet paper, cater to our needs. Our dollars matter and we can spend them wisely.

"A wise man once gave me this piece of advice: 'The more you give, the more you live.' I hope to be running TOMS for the rest of my life, and to one day give millions of shoes away to millions of kids!"

FIVE THINGS YOU CAN DO NOW

1. Throw a Style Your Sole party: Buy your TOMS shoes and get together with a group of friends and some fabric paint, glitter, stencils, whatever, to customize them. You'll get exactly what you want and provide a gift for others, too. This is a great way to raise awareness among friends and family.

2. Search out companies that make the world a better place. How you spend your dollars matters. Use this power wisely.

Buy products that are working to bring about environmental and social change.

3. As much as possible, buy products made from organic cotton or other natural/sustainable fibers such as wool and hemp. The cultivation of conventional cotton is devastating to the environment and uses more pesticides than any other crop in the world.

4. Buy vintage and preworn clothes. Having style does not have to mean spending a ton of money; it is about having the courage to express your own unique identity. Going vintage shopping is one of my favorite things in the world.

5. Get as much life out of your clothes as possible. When I am through with my TOMS, they are downright nasty.

When you're choosing your kids' clothes, try to avoid the temptation to give in to their "desperate" need for mall majors like Limited Too, Abercrombie, and American Eagle. Try to enlist their compassion and acquiescence by discussing the building of brands, the cost associated with the saturation of advertising (tens of thousands of dollars just for the ad space in magazines—plus models' and photographers' fees), and what that does to the ticket price of the garment they are pining for in the store. It's great to feel good about how you look, but it's also important—in fact, perhaps most important—to arm our kids with the knowledge that helps them discern why they want what (they think) they want. After all, we only hold the purse strings for a few short years.

WHEN YOU DO BUY

• Choose quality over trends.

• Opt for natural fibers.

• Organic is best, not just for food. Organic cotton, organic wool, and even organic silk are all available in greater supply than ever.

• Skip anything that is "dry-clean only." It'll burn through carbon emissions, and your wallet, pretty quickly.

• Launder on cold all the time, to save loads of energy.

• Hang to dry whenever feasible. You'll save about a hundred dollars a year, reduce your carbon emissions, and extend the life of your garments.

YOU ARE WHAT YOU WEAR 2: THE OTHER STUFF YOU'RE DONNING

A touch of color for your cheeks, a bit of gloss for your lips. It's a pick-me-up few women can resist. But when you choose cosmetics or fragrance, in many ways you really *are* what you wear. In fact, you're ingesting it so much you might as well be eating it. Unbelievable as it may sound, most of the ingredients in shampoos, body lotions, mascaras, and lipsticks are not tested for safety. And I don't mean only the ones at your local drugstore, either; this includes the really swanky ones gleaming under glass at the big department stores, too. There is just no regulatory government body overseeing these prettifying concoctions. A whopping eighty-nine percent of the thousands of chemical ingredients in cosmetics come to market without any testing.

It's really time for us to rethink what we're putting on our bodies. Because in the case of cosmetics, if we're putting them on, we're putting them in. And in case you think I'm exaggerating, just remember the nicotine patch.

When it comes to body care, many of us worked to keep our babies safe by using organic baby products; well, the same goes for our growing kids! Experts say sixty percent of ingredients can be absorbed in our skin. This is especially an issue for younger kids, because their bodies are different from adults'. They don't sweat as much as adults, and this means that they are not as efficient at eliminating toxins as adults, so we need to be even more vigilant about their exposure.

Meet a couple of Green Gurus doing everything in their power to protect you and your family from these largely unaddressed dangers.

Green Guru

Jeremiah McElwee
GLOBAL WHOLE BODY COORDINATOR,
WHOLE FOODS MARKET
DAD

For the past two years Jeremiah has worked to develop and implement a clear set of standards for cosmetics and body care in an industry that has been largely unregulated. He helped pen the Whole Foods Market Premium Body Care

Standard, which he told me he did to make a safer, better world for his two young daughters.

"We always think about what we eat and how important that is, and obviously that's what we are all about at Whole Foods Market—how it affects your health and well-being. Today we're also finding more and more science showing that what you put on your body is just as important, because it gets absorbed into your skin.

"The skin is the largest detoxification organ in the body. Whatever you're putting on your body can enter through your pores, especially in the shower. You are way more apt to absorb chemicals into your body under those conditions. The heat, steam, and water open you up. As you're lathering your body and washing your hair, it's a prime time for chemicals to be entering.

"So what are you 'wearing'? What are you ingesting? Chances are, it's chemicals from all kinds of products: lotions, body butters, deodorants, cosmetics, soaps, and shampoos. They enter your bloodstream and have to be cleaned by the liver, too.

"For this reason, at Whole Foods Market we decided to eliminate confusion about what is safe. We've established clear ingredient standards for every product. It's called the Premium Body Care Standard. In the past there was no definition for 'natural' and so everyone's really been able to use that term on any product they wanted. Customers assumed they were getting clean, safe, eco-friendly, earth-friendly products. But the reality is, they were buying into a marketing pitch. There's no governmental standard and no industry standard, so we felt we had to step up and clarify: What is safe? What is green? What is clean?

"For a product to meet our new standards, it must contain no artificial colors or preservatives. We went through every ingredient in every product on our shelves and asked, is this the safest option available based on published safety data?

"The result? The cleanest and most eco-friendly products in the world.

"You don't have to read labels when you buy food at Whole Foods Market, and we wanted our customers to have the same experience when buying other products."

Red Flag

Anything containing parabens, synthetic fragrances, and FD&C colors—some of these are known as coal tar colors.

Green Flag

• Aubrey Organics kids' shampoo (no eye sting—and my daughter Mina is VERY sensitive)

• Good old citronella essential oil for insects

• Dr. Hauschka sunscreen (smells great and goes on clean, not messy)

• Natural Dentist toothpaste (kids' and adults' both work great and are sodium lauryl sulfate free)

• Depth body washes (they smell and feel great on the skin)

THE BIG THREE

When kids get older, there are three biggies to keep your eye on: makeup, deodorant, and hair dye.

First of all, even though it may be hard for us to accept, there comes a time when our little girls will be asking to buy makeup. Knowing the questionable ingredients that are prominent in conventional makeup lines, I have been thankful to have all-natural choices available. This is a perfect example of starting off right, meaning choosing natural ingredients and initiating that healthy habit for the rest of their lives. My favorites, though pricey, are Dr. Hauschka, Zia, and Mineral Fusion. I know my daughters are not getting any extra EA (estrogenic activity) to flip-flop their already raging hormones.

The second one to monitor is deodorant. Most conventional products are not just deodorants—i.e., designed to mask the smell of sweat—but antiperspirants, designed to shut off the sweat glands. That's just not natural! Sweating is one of the body's crucial paths for getting rid of toxins. Do not buy anything that contains the controversial aluminum-based antiperspirant ingredients, which may have harmful health effects. The most natural choice? A salt stick. It may have to be applied a couple of times a day, but it does no harm and, for at least a few hours, does the trick. You can drop one in the gym bag to be reapplied after exercise.

Third, many kids, both boys and girls, have an almost hypnotic desire to color their hair as they hit the teens. But beware: Twenty-two potentially carcinogenic hair-dye chemicals that have been banned in the European Union are still used in some U.S. dyes. If you use a home dye, check the ingredients for Acid Orange 24 and 2,3-naphthalenediol; these are some of the most toxic chemicals.

Green Guru

Erin Schrode

SIXTEEN-YEAR-OLD ACTRESS, MODEL AND GREEN GIRL
FOUNDING MEMBER, TEENS FOR SAFE COSMETICS

Erin is one of those rare kids who has it all. She's really smart, ridiculously beautiful, fit, healthy, and honestly nice. But the really amazing thing about Erin is she has already found her raison d'être. She knows things aren't quite right in our world, and she's doing what she can to change them. With a spoonful of her organic sugar, who could possibly say no? In fact, because of Erin and her young buddies at Teens for Safe Cosmetics, and their relentless visits to Governor Schwarzenegger's office last year, California became the first state to pass the Toxic Toys Act. Now the state of California has got toxic toiletries on their agenda, and we'll all be safer because of it.

"This is all we have—one world, one body—but here we are, abusing both! This kind of denial and avoidance is not an option anymore. We are feeling the direct effects of our actions right now. People are getting sick; global warming is happening; forests are being cut down; water is contaminated. Everything is a mess and we wonder why. We're looking for the cure, but we should be searching for the cause.

"What you do now is vital. We can work together for a better place to live and a safer and healthier body.

"What you eat, what's in your home, what you put on your body—it all matters. You can only control so much, but what you *can* do, you *should*. What you are wearing on your body is absorbed into your bloodstream and affects your health. When you shampoo, condition, moisturize, or brush your teeth, you're introducing chemicals into your body—and lots of them. If you're a woman, you probably use between fifteen and twenty-five cosmetic products a day, a total of hundreds of different chemicals, many of which have proven links to cancer, birth defects, and reproductive harm. Frankly, that's not something that I want to put on my body.

"Unlike food or pharmaceuticals, cosmetics are not monitored by any federal body—the FDA requires no testing. The companies do not even have to disclose exactly what is in their products. They can say 'fragrance' or 'our secret blend.'

"Don't worry, you don't have to stop being clean and beautiful! There are loads of companies out there making amazing products that are clean, green, and organic.

"When I have kids, I want them to grow up in a world where they don't have to worry that people aren't doing right by the planet, where they know that everything around them has been made in a thoughtful, mindful way—where they can feel good about going to the store and not worry about the ethics of what they are buying."

FIVE THINGS THAT YOU CAN GO OUT AND DO TOMORROW

1. Become an informed consumer. Learn about the effects of a product on the body and the environment. Read labels and pay attention to ingredients, packaging, origin, manufacturing practices, and any other information you can glean.

2. Bring your own bag to the grocery store. These are not only reusable but often larger and easier to carry than a typical throwaway bag.

3. Swap one of your cosmetic or personal-care products for a greener alternative. Switch just one item and you are already making a difference.

4. Buy locally. Not only will you have an idea of where the products are coming from, but you will also conserve a lot of resources, including petroleum!

5. As eloquently stated by Reese Witherspoon's character in *Legally Blonde*, "Speak up, America, speak up!" Find a cause that excites you and join the movement.

YOU ARE WHAT YOU BUY: I WANT THAT!

I love stuff. Maybe you do, too. As a culture, we Americans *really* love our stuff. We are about 3.5 percent of the world's population, but we consume about 26 percent of the world's gross domestic product (WGDP).

In case you think we're about to take a guilt trip down the conspicuous-consumption road, don't you fret. I'm here to tell you to keep loving your stuff. Although I may not be the most popular person in the community co-op, and I risk possibly being banned from the ashram, I still gotta call 'em as I see 'em: *Reduce, Reuse, Recycle* is good, but *Rethink, Reward, Rework* is even better.

Let's *Rethink* what we're doing with our stuff, and take into consideration,

- Where does it come from?

- Who made it?

- Who touched it?

- Under what conditions?

- What will happen to it when I'm done?

Let's *Reward* the manufacturers, stores, and companies that support our communities by offering ethical, sustainable, earth- and people-friendly goods and services.

Let's *Rework* anything that we like to buy that is taking a heavy toll on the environment. Earth matters. We simply can't afford to pretend it doesn't anymore. (What's the alternative for our kids' future—living on the moon?)

Green Guru

Priya Haji
**CEO AND COFOUNDER, WORLD OF GOOD,
FAIR TRADE GIFTS AND ACCESSORIES**

I've met Priya many times and I consider her a good friend. We came into this new time, this renaissance called the green movement, from different corners, mine environmental and hers sociological, but it takes four corners to form a strong base. And fair trade is not a folksy feel-good standard for us to consider, but a way to equalize the playing field and em- brace that indeed there is enough for us all. Priya is making sure of that on her end, and besides that, she's a one-stop shop for the memorable, beautiful gifts I give to my friends and family.

"Our company mission is to make it really easy to buy things in a way that makes life better for the people who make those things.

"It isn't about buying more or less; it's about buying differently. Choose fair trade and you can make the world a better place.

"What does fair trade mean? It means the person who made the product was paid fairly, and had good working conditions. No child labor. Fair trade means there were local leaders and local nonprofits monitoring that.

"Fair trade is the idea that when we engage in free trade, we think about the people behind the products we're buying. In the same way that organic food has gotten us to think about what is in our food, fair trade asks us to think about who makes our products. In the global supply chain, it's usually the laborers physically making the products who are paid the least. With fair trade, we make sure the producer receives a fair percentage of the total. In the end, fair trade will only work if we as consumers choose to purchase products made in an ethical way. We have tremendous power as consumers to shape the way the world does business. Fair trade ensures that everyone is treated with dignity and respect and that is a great investment.

"Of all the great products we offer at World of Good, one of my favorites is from a cooperative in Africa called 'Gone

Rural,' an organization working with women in an area where the HIV infection rates are very high. These women collect grass and weave amazingly beautiful boxes and baskets and lunch boxes. Many of these women are supporting not only their children but the AIDS orphans in the community, too.

"So choosing one of these amazing baskets, to store your magazines in or hold fruit in the center of your dining table, can enrich not just your life but many lives. It just makes sense to me.

"Every day, I feel very lucky to have the opportunity to work together to build a new vision of commerce—where the products themselves are the source of good things in the world. Last year World of Good worked with 142 artisan groups in 34 countries. I think we are unlocking a new future."

WHAT FAIR TRADE MEANS

You can't monitor the business practices of all the companies in the world, but your purchasing power is one of the strongest weapons you have, and you should do some due diligence before you open up your pocketbook. World of Good has a very helpful checklist.

COMPANIES THAT FOLLOW FAIR TRADE PRACTICES

• Pay a fair wage to the artisan. Check the Fair Wage Guide at www.fairtradecalculator.net to see what a fair price is in the local context.

- Purchase from cooperatives, nonprofit organizations, or directly from the artisans whenever possible. If using an intermediary, ensure that a fair portion goes back to the artisan.

- Provide employment without discrimination, and strive to create employment opportunities for women and the most disadvantaged communities.

- Ensure that all artisans have access to a safe and clean work environment, whether it is a workshop, a community meeting space, or their own homes.

- Guarantee that no child labor is used in production—unless the entire family is involved in the craft and the children are still attending school.

- Follow environmentally sustainable production practices whenever possible: Encourage artisans to select local raw materials, harvest them sustainably, and use renewable energy. Avoid processes that require artificial chemicals.

- Maintain business practices that are open to public scrutiny, and make every effort to be as transparent as possible.

IN THE BAG

Paper, plastic, or organic? It's not just what you're putting in the bag but the bag itself that makes a HUGE difference.

If you're a family of four shopping for groceries, chances are, you use at least 12 plastic bags a week. Times 52 weeks, that's 624 plastic bags a year for your family alone (and that doesn't even count the trips to the drugstore, deli, or bookstore)!!

We can either be Conscious Consumers (thank you, beautiful Katie Lee Joel, for explaining that to me!) or we are stuck being Unconscious Consumers.

In the U.S. alone we use one hundred billion plastic bags a year. One hundred billion bags, each of which takes a thousand years to decompose in a landfill! As if that's not bad enough, bags fly and float everywhere and tens of thousands of marine animals are strangled every year as they mistake floating plastic bags for jellyfish. No one wants to be a part of that, and together we can make a huge difference, and some companies and stores make that choice especially easy.

Green Guru

Sharon Rowe
FOUNDER, ECO-BAGS
MOM

I have known Green Guru Sharon Rowe for over ten years. I can tell you for sure she is the real deal, a super-green pioneer. Two decades ago she founded Eco-Bags because she was keyed in (a good bit ahead of most of us) to the huge waste that comes with plastic-bag consumption.

"I started in 1989, the year my son was born. It was my own reaction to all the plastic bags that I was using at my neighborhood stores. Every day I was bringing home plastic bags, and I also saw them everywhere—in gutters, stuck in trees, and blowing around like big puffy leaves or strange dirty ghosts. They were making things a mess! I felt bad just throwing them away, but I had a tiny New York City kitchen, so storing them was silly.

"I decided I wanted to bring my own bags, like I saw people doing when I was traveling in Europe, but I couldn't find any. I thought, if I'm interested, I bet other people are, too. I found a great source in India and started the Web site.

"It changed me in so many ways. The bag is the baby step. When you bring your own bag to the store, it changes your relationship to shopping. I started to see the strangeness of putting wastefully packaged foods into my Eco-Bags, and it made me consider every purchase more carefully. I began looking for pure food. It was part of making me conscious of what I was feeding my child.

"The bag keeps you in your moment—and begins so many conversations at checkout. 'Why are you doing that? Where did you get that?' It turns a trip to the grocery store into a social outing. And that's a practice I really want to engage in—it is a very loving thing.

"It's kind of an easy choice—cleaning up the planet one bag at a time. That one simple gesture multiplied by millions of people can make a huge impact in the world."

YOU ARE WHAT YOU DO: LIVE WELL

For some of us, what we do for a living doesn't define us; it's the means to an end, or the paycheck that allows us to relax and hang out with family and friends. But for others, what they do is a huge part of the heartbeat of who they are. This is especially true for the pioneers and visionaries of the green movement. Here are two remarkably different Green Gurus who personify the power of one.

Green Guru

Deborah Koons Garcia
FILMMAKER
ENVIRONMENTALIST

Oh, the popcorn, the plush seats, the hush that falls over the kids as the lights dim ... we are ready to be amused, enlightened, and entertained by a great film. Deborah Koons Garcia at Lily Films has made one of the most applauded and informative documentaries of our time, *The Future of Food*. An unforgettable exploration of genetic engineering in our food supply, it does for GE what Al Gore's *An Inconvenient Truth* does for global warming....It enables you to "get it." How lucky for us she has turned her lens there. Now she's working on the more upbeat but equally mind-altering doc *In Good Heart Soil*, about the mystery of fertility.

"We are part of the soil community and we cannot ignore that. There are no high-tech fixes: If we ignore the soil, we can't grow food; if soil is abused and exploited, we can't grow food. That's why we are sick.

"Today there are two different ways of looking at agriculture. The corporate/chemical and the organic/sustainable.

Sixty years ago corporations pushed into agriculture because they had so many chemicals left over from World War II; plus a lot of people really believed it would drive up yield, and it did. But it also wears out the soil—chemically-dependent agriculture takes and takes and takes.

"I want to help people understand that we need to re-think how we grow food. Chemical agriculture is totally dependent on oil. Pesticides and herbicides are made from petroleum. Huge machinery is used to manage these enormous farms. Then crops are shipped thousands of miles.

"As we choose to power down and use less energy, we need to eat more locally. The future could be really nice, with delicious locally grown food, less consumerism. But if we don't do it consciously, the change will be abrupt, a crisis in the world where people, even very affluent people, could literally starve.

"One of the other things I think would be great is if people started to focus on the quality of life, not the quantity. We need to cut back on all the consumerism we are all so addicted to. How can we use our time in a way that is not material? Instead of using your time to go shopping, use your time to go for a walk with a friend. Instead of going to hang out at the mall, go to a friend's house and make a really nice meal or play a game. I think we need to feed what gives us a sense of real peace:

• Having a garden

• A conversation

• Being with our families

• The nonmaterial is what we need to connect with

"We need to recognize that nature has its own wisdom; it has its own life. The earth has its own integrity; when we respect it, we can live happily and healthily. We need to do the same with ourselves. We have the right to respect the integrity of our kids by not being pulled to buy things that are bad for them. We need to find out what qualities we can foster in ourselves to strengthen our own sense of integrity, courage, discernment.

"I believe we all really do have purpose, a calling, if you will. Sometimes connecting with ours happens by chance, an almost supernatural bolt of lightning. Sometimes it is just the yearning and desire to better the soulful aspect of our lives. Either way, I want to encourage you to connect to your purpose, the message that you are meant to experience and deliver."

Sound lofty? Consider this: Our next Green Guru, called one of the greatest orators of our time, came upon her calling following her shelter mutt through a junkyard. Hey, if she can find, and help create, paradise there, what gems do we have in our own backyards? I think there are many. . . .

Green Guru

Majora Carter
FOUNDER AND EXECUTIVE DIRECTOR,
SUSTAINABLE SOUTH BRONX
URBAN-REVITALIZATION SPECIALIST

This beautiful and gifted young woman is a conduit of light for us and for our children. She's a visionary who has the power to entrance us with her dream. To hear Majora speak is to be in the presence of greatness (and now that you've read the whole book, you know I don't say that lightly). We are so lucky fate or happenstance put her in our here and now, because, for sure, anywhere she is, is much the better for her presence. Take a gander at how she came to be today's Joan of Arc . . . knowing the way, and leading us all forward. . . .

"I moved back home to the South Bronx in the late nineties. I became part of a community of artists, and around that time we discovered that the city and state were planning to build a huge waste facility in the middle of our residential neighborhood. Now, the South Bronx already processes about forty percent of the municipal waste for the city of New York and this would bring another forty percent—just tons and tons of waste. We already had a sewage sludge processing plant using all kinds of chemicals, and the smell is just awful for blocks and blocks.

"I was just a regular person, but when I realized we were carrying a disproportionate toxic burden, I became political.

I decided I wanted to be part of the solution. We needed more sustainable waste management.

"We went out to the community to see how they felt. People were alarmed that the company contracted to build the plant was not going to be able to go in so gently or with such environmental care as they said, and it was going to most affect those of us who live here. This is our home.

"After you know what you don't want, it's important to focus on what you do want. So we started a community visioning process—it wasn't what I came up with, but the community. They wanted

• clean air

• parks within walking distance

• transportation that worked for them, more routes to where they lived

• living-wage jobs that didn't degrade the environment

"We managed to keep the toxic waste plant out of our community, and we did more than that. We ended up with a beautiful park that families will enjoy for generations. This vision began to take shape thanks to my dog, Xena. One day while I was out jogging with her, she took me into this old abandoned junkyard, a dump. At that time we had a few in the area. Amazingly, through the dump, at the end, was this beautiful, amazing waterfront: the Bronx River.

"I went back to my apartment and wrote a proposal for

seed money to begin to revitalize that specific stretch of land. Our goal was to create a park on that site so people could have access to this beautiful river. I wasn't ashamed to ask for help. Actually, I was surprised when someone said no. But I wasn't going to be stopped by someone else's foolishness just because they couldn't understand a great idea.

"Four years, and a lot of volunteer hours and grants later, we ended up opening that park. Last year I got married there.

"Most people have no idea how much their interest is often aligned with other people who they might think are not like them at all.

"The world would be a much sweeter place if none of us had to fight for crumbs and we understood we all have the capacity to make much bigger pies. And it's right within our grasp, this sense of community."

WE ARE THE WORLD

When our kids were tiny babies, zonked out snug in our arms or gurgling in our laps, we had tremendous power—the ability to make their world a wonderful, nurturing place. Our arms may not be big enough to hold them now, and goodness knows, I can't bounce any of my kids on my knees these days, but I've still got the power. I've learned to expand my safe haven for my kids' sake (and all our kids' sake).

Me and you, we are the world, and our safe havens can stretch up to the highest mountaintops and down to the deepest riverbeds. Our voices can be heard on the school playground, and in the boardrooms of Fortune 500 companies.

We have an unprecedented opportunity to do what every parent in every generation all across the world wants: to make a better way for our kids.

We're all in this together—in fact, we're all *on* this together. We're connected in ways as fluid and powerful as the sea. We choose whom we vote for, what we buy, support, and use. The buck has stopped here, and it's great to be the boss.

Because one by one, we make all the difference in the world.

I'm very grateful that you've let me join you for a little while. And thank you for meeting my wonderful Green Gurus. I hope they've given you some ideas you can put to use for your own family.

Remember: Turning green is not a duty; it's a right. You have the right to clean water, fresh air, and transparency in terms of the products you use and buy, and most of all you have the right to vibrant health for you and your family.

Go for the Green, and enjoy those wonderful kids.

GREEN AT A GLANCE

 Evergreen: Commit your waking hours to the big picture, a way to sustain the planet, a green economy, and your community.

Pea green: Put the power of your consumerism to work for what you believe in and want; be a conscious consumer.

Spring green: Consider changing your diet to be more locally season specific. At least two nights a week, "eat local," preferably—at least partially—from your own backyard.

Green Goods

To find out more about the wonderful people and organizations you've read about in the book:

One

IPM, integrated pest management
Fact sheets and info from the EPA.
www.epa.gov/opp00001/factsheets/ipm.htm

Beyond Pesticides
The most helpful, comprehensive site on this subject on the Web.
www.beyondpesticides.org

Centers for Disease Control
Scary stats on pesticide exposure and helpful tips on integrated pest management and avoiding exposure.
www.cdc.gov

Sierra Club
America's oldest and largest environmental organization. Their

motto: "*Explore, enjoy, and protect the planet.*" *Membership has perks, too.*
www.sierraclub.org

Worldwide Orphans Foundation
Check out what they are doing for kids who don't have loving moms and dads to look out for them—innovative programs that do much more than save lives.
www.wwo.org

Grassroots Healthy Lawn Program
Easy tips for a great green lawn.
www.ghlp.org

Waterkeeper Alliance
The umbrella nonprofit that keeps rivers, lakes, and well water clean in hundreds of chapters around the world.
www.waterkeeper.org

Garden Tykes
Some nice garden-inspired things.
www.gardentykes.com
908-692-6316

Planet Natural
Fantastic site with friendly, knowledgeable staff to help you get your green thumb on! You can order wonderful hungry insects, too!
www.planetnatural.com
800-289-6656

Two

Newman's Own
Peruse the mouthwatering offerings and find fun recipes, too. Remember, they are GIVING away all the profits.
www.newmansown.com

Environmental Defense Fund
Many, many helpful downloadable lists that make safe eco-shopping really easy.
www.edf.org

Center for Science in the Public Interest
Since 1971, the Center for Science in the Public Interest has been a strong advocate for nutrition, health, and food safety. Check out their list of the ten best and worst foods.
www.cspinet.org

The Feingold Association
A membership-driven organization working to reduce food allergies and sensitivities in the hundreds of thousands of affected individuals. Check out their symptoms list.
www.feingold.org
Feingold Association of the United States
554 East Main Street Suite 301
Riverhead, NY 11901
800-321-3287 (U.S. only)

Greens Restaurant
Chef Annie Somerville's famous vegetarian restaurant. An amazing experience in a beautiful locale.

Building A, Fort Mason Center
San Francisco, CA 94123
415-771-6222

AllergyKids
Great downloadable steps of what you can do at the grocery store, in your kids' school, etc.
www.allergykids.com

Farmer Steve's
Simply the world's best popcorn and no GMOs.
www.farmersteve.com

Three

The Nature Conservancy
They have a great carbon calculator on the site.
www.nature.org
4245 North Fairfax Drive
Suite 100
Arlington, VA 22203-1606
703-841-5300

Natural Spaces Domes
One of the leading manufacturers of geodesic dome homes. They also offer a hands-on Dome School.
www.naturalspacesdomes.com
37955 Bridge Road
North Branch, MN 55056
1-800-733-7107

Marcal

Pretty much the original high-recycled-content household paper products. Available almost everywhere.

www.marcalpaper.com

Whole Foods

The world's largest and most innovative natural and organic grocery store. The Web site now has lively and fun podcasts, too.

www.wholefoods.com

Seventh Generation

The grandfather of "green clean," founder Jeffrey Hollender is a true pioneer. In thousands of stores, on Amazon.com and www. seventhgeneration.com.

Green Depot

All things green for home improvement. They started to service the chemically sensitive, but the rest of us can benefit from their nontoxic expertise, as well.

www.greendepot.com

Cheryl Terrace's Vital Design design studio

www.vitaldesignltd.com

212-799-1540

Craigslist

Search by city for all kinds of cool stuff, some of it totally free!

www.craigslist.org

Four

ReusableBags.com
A huge selection of fabric goody bags and all sorts of other reusable bags.
www.reusablebags.com

Garden Harvest
Fun, wonderful organization that lets you donate live farm animals to rural families in need.
www.gardenharvest.org

budget101.com/hw1.htm
Great costume ideas.

Dr. Hauschka
The best, cleanest body care and makeup.
Available at all Whole Foods and www.drhauschka.com.

Aubrey Organics
Very clean makeup and body-care products.
www.aubreyorganics.com

Original Good
The part of World of Good where you can purchase their cool fair trade collection of gifts and housewares. Some of the nicest handbags on the planet, too.
www.originalgood.com

Global Exchange
Wonderful international human rights organization with lots of fas-

cinating info online, but a great store for fair trade goods, too.
www.globalexchange.org

Ten Thousand Villages
Brick-and-mortar stores across the U.S. and Canada where you can find everything from folk art and heirloom-quality home decor to ceramics, textiles, baskets, jewelry, and musical instruments. Shop online or check the store locator to see if you're near one.
www.tenthousandvillages.com

Heifer International
Donate an animal (or contribute to the donation of one) to a village in need.
www.heifer.org
1 World Avenue
Little Rock, AR 72202
800-422-0474

ecobusinesslinks.com/organic_christmas_trees
Organic Christmas-tree finder.

Organic Bouquet
Organic centerpieces or wreaths.
www.organicbouquet.com

Big Dipper Wax Works
More great beeswax candles.
www.bigdipperwaxworks.com

Five

Church Street School for Music and Art

Wonderful art and music school in lower Manhattan with ongoing events open to the public.
www.churchstreetschool.org
74 Warren Street
New York, NY 10007
212-571-7290

John Wargo

Professor of environmental risk analysis and policy, and political science, Yale University; child welfare advocate; and author of environment-changing books including Our Children's Toxic Legacy: How Science and Law Fail to Protect Us from Pesticides *and* Taking Control: Health, Environmental Quality, and Individual Freedom.

Kids for Saving Earth

Tessa Hill's powerful nonprofit, founded by her heroic son, Clint. Lots of fun stuff to help our kids save the earth.
www.kidsforsavingearth.org

Go Green Initiative

A program that works to create a culture of environmental responsibility on school campuses throughout the United States. Includes tips for teachers and parents.
www.gogreeninitiative.org

Six

school-lunch.org
Great information on food dyes and additives and links to the Feingold Diet.

Better School Food
Dr. Susan Rubin's comprehensive site suggests ways to circumvent the worst of the bad stuff in the lunch line, and strategies to remove it forever. Very helpful lists to download.
www.betterschoolfood.org

angrymoms.org
Amy Kalafa's site based on her documentary film Two Angry Moms, *but also a call to arms and connections if you decide you want to step up and lead the fight.*

foodnavigator.com
Lists of specific ingredients and what they really mean.

Wrap-N-Mat
My favorite alternative to plastic sandwich bags—but go for the PVC free, natch.
www.wrap-n-mat.com

Seven

Back to Basics Toys
Great toys and games that are, indeed, back to basics.
www.backtobasicstoys.com

woodentoys.com

A huge selection—may be the world's largest selection—of wooden toys. And wood is good.

Toys "R" Us

Now they've done it! They've stepped up and introduced an FSC-certified line of unfinished wooden toys. They are shipped from China, but still, they start at only $9.99 and they're really nice! Available at all Toys "R" Us nationwide and www.toysrus.com.

PlanetGreen.com

Cool, craftsy do-it-yourself stuff is often blogged here. (I write for them, too.)

WorstedWitch.com

Jasmin Malik Chua's wildly imaginative craft site.

Eight

American Academy of Pediatrics

Sometimes staunchly old-school, they still have strong recommendations and backup about strategies for reducing TV that you may find helpful.
www.aap.org

PBS

The original home of safe TV, Mr. Rogers, Sesame Street, *and Mr. Purple himself (no, not Prince—Barney!). Pretty wonderful stuff, in moderation, and for the younger set.*
www.pbs.org

Discovery Channel
*Both the mother ship and its spin-off Planet Green offer great
how-to television and Web content. Also the new home of Emeril,
Ed Begley Jr., and the wonderful Sara Snow. Check local listings.*
www.dsc.discovery.com

National Geographic
*The magazine and the television channel are both especially good for
families with older kids.*
www.nationalgeographic.com

Nine

Think bars
www.thinkproducts.com

Dr. Susan Rubin
www.drsusanrubin.com

TOMS Shoes
www.tomsshoes.com

Teens for Safe Cosmetics
*These girls will make you feel GREAT about the next generation!
Maybe it is all going to be OK. . . .*
www.teensforsafecosmetics.org

WorldofGoodInc.com
*An online community all about fair trade and our connection to one
another through the goods we purchase.*

Eco-Bags
The original reusable bag.
www.ecobags.com

Deborah Koons Garcia
The Future of Food *is her highly entertaining and startling film on genetic engineering in our food supply. Today's version of* Silent Spring.
www.lilyfilms.com

Sustainable South Bronx
Learn what one woman can do to take desolate wasteland and turn it into something beautiful for all of us to enjoy. Talk about the power of the human spirit!
www.ssbx.org

(This page constitutes an extension of the copyright page:)

Photos on pages 1 and 3 by H. Fassa.
Photos on pages 33, 97, 121, 145, 169, 193 and 207 by
Mina Fassa.
Photos on pages 71 and 171 by Linda Skoog.
Photo on page 99 by Will Paradise.